COPING WITH CANDIDA
Are yeast infections draining your energy?

SHIRLEY TRICKETT trained as a nurse before becoming a counsellor and teacher. She is the author of *Irritable Bowel Syndrome and Diverticulosis* (Thorsons 1999, new edition). Her other books include *Coming off Tranquillisers and Sleeping Pills* (Thorsons 1987), *Coping with Anxiety and Depression* (Sheldon 1989) and *Coping Successfully with Panic Attacks* (Sheldon 1992). In 1987 she won a Whitbread Community Care Award.

D0308406

Overcoming Common Problems Series

For a full list of titles please contact
Sheldon Press, Marylebone Road, London NW1 4DU

Antioxidants
DR ROBERT YOUNGSON

The Assertiveness Workbook
A plan for busy women
JOANNA GUTMANN

Beating the Comfort Trap
DR WINDY DRYDEN AND JACK
GORDON

Birth Over Thirty Five
SHEILA KITZINGER

Body Language
How to read others' thoughts by their
gestures
ALLAN PEASE

Body Language in Relationships
DAVID COHEN

Calm Down
How to cope with frustration and anger
DR PAUL HAUCK

Cancer – A Family Affair
NEVILLE SHONE

The Cancer Guide for Men
HELEN BEARE AND NEIL PRIDDY

The Candida Diet Book
KAREN BRODY

Caring for Your Elderly Parent
JULIA BURTON-JONES

Cider Vinegar
MARGARET HILLS

Comfort for Depression
JANET HORWOOD

Coping Successfully with Hayfever
DR ROBERT YOUNGSON

**Coping Successfully with Joint
Replacement**
DR TOM SMITH

Coping Successfully with Migraine
SUE DYSON

Coping Successfully with Pain
NEVILLE SHONE

Coping Successfully with Panic Attacks
SHIRLEY TRICKETT

Coping Successfully with PMS
KAREN EVENNETT

**Coping Successfully with Prostate
Problems**
ROSY REYNOLDS

**Coping Successfully with Your Hiatus
Hernia**
DR TOM SMITH

**Coping Successfully with Your Irritable
Bladder**
JENNIFER HUNT

**Coping Successfully with Your Irritable
Bowel**
ROSEMARY NICOL

Coping with Anxiety and Depression
SHIRLEY TRICKETT

Coping with Blushing
DR ROBERT EDELMANN

Coping with Breast Cancer
DR EADIE HEYDERMAN

Coping with Bronchitis and Emphysema
DR TOM SMITH

Coping with Candida
SHIRLEY TRICKETT

Coping with Chronic Fatigue
TRUDIE CHALDER

Coping with Coeliac Disease
KAREN BRODY

Coping with Cystitis
CAROLINE CLAYTON

Coping with Depression and Elation
DR PATRICK McKEON

Coping with Eczema
DR ROBERT YOUNGSON

Coping with Endometriosis
JO MEARS

Coping with Fibroids
MARY-CLAIRE MASON

Coping with Headaches
SHIRLEY TRICKETT

Coping with a Hernia
DR DAVID DELVIN

Coping with Psoriasis
PROFESSOR RONALD MARKS

Coping with Rheumatism and Arthritis
DR ROBERT YOUNGSON

Overcoming Common Problems Series

Overcoming Common Problems Series

Overcoming Common Problems

COPING WITH CANDIDA

*Are yeast infections draining
your energy?*

Shirley Trickett

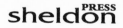

First published in Great Britain in 1994 by
Sheldon Press, SPCK, Marylebone Road, London NW1 4DU

Fourth impression 1999

British Library Cataloguing-in-Publication Data
A catalogue record for this book is available from the British Library
ISBN 0–85969–688–X

Photoset by Deltatype Ltd, Ellesmere Port, Cheshire
Printed in Great Britain by Biddles Ltd, Guildford and King's Lynn

For my friends and teachers
Elizabeth and Keith Thompson
with love and gratitude

Contents

Acknowledgements

Thank you to my friend Ann Marie Curry for providing the information on aerobics in Chapter 8, and for her love.

Apologies to my son, David, who was unfortunate enough to be staying with me whilst I wrote this book, and had to suffer 'candida talk' with breakfast, lunch and dinner.

Introduction

You could have picked up this book thinking 'What on earth is Candida', or you might have chosen it because you suffer from repeated attacks of thrush and know that this is the organism responsible for the condition. Or it might be that you have battled for years with chronic problems and are looking for answers as to why your 'irritable bowel' does not respond to conventional treatment, why you have food and chemical intolerances, why you suffer chronic fatigue, why you cannot lose weight on a calorie-controlled diet, why you crave sweet or yeasty foods, why you have thrush before every period, why your PMT is getting worse, why you have mood swings and other psychological symptoms. These are all problems that can be due to an overgrowth of candida in the bowel.

It is true that many of the above problems have their origin in conditions other than candida and it would be unwise to act hastily before you have consulted your doctor. If on the other hand your symptoms have been investigated and you have not had satisfactory answers then it would be worthwhile looking at the list of predisposing factors (particularly if you have been on long-term antibiotics) and also seeing how you score on the candida questionnaire.

What is candida?

Candida is a yeast which is normally present in the bowel. It feeds on the simple carbohydrates we eat such as sugar, bread, biscuits, cakes and fermented foods such as cheese, alcohol and vinegar. If the immune system is healthy the growth of the candida can be kept under control; if it is not healthy, having been weakened by some prescribed drugs, such as antibiotics or steroids, or if resistance is low through poor nutrition, excessive alcohol, stress, illness or pollution, then the yeast can grow to such an extent that it interferes with normal body chemistry and can cause widespread baffling symptoms.

1

Is candida just the 'in thing' to have?

Sceptics have said of people with chronic candida problems that they read too many magazine health articles; people love lists of symptoms; candida is just the malady of the moment – a whitewash for hypochondrias and neurotic symptoms. Perhaps those who are not willing to look at the possibility of candida overgrowth causing chronic health problems should look at the alarming increase of anti-yeast prescriptions, even over the past ten years; they might ask themselves why, if the problem does not exist, there is a need for candida help-lines and support groups and, most importantly, why these patients lose all their 'neurotic' symptoms when they are correctly diagnosed and receive the appropriate treatment: anti-fungal preparations and dietary adjustments.

The content of this book

This book describes what an overgrowth of candida can do to the body; how it can produce conditions which range from minor irritations to severe debilitating physical and psychological illness. It discusses the causal factors and who is most likely to be at risk. It also highlights why so many people are affected and why there is a division of medical opinion on the subject. More importantly, from your point of view, the following pages should enable you to decide whether your long-investigated symptoms arise from an overgrowth of fungus and, happily, what you can safely do about it. It seeks not only to give clear suggestions on how to control candida with safe anti-fungal preparations, diet and nutritional supplements, but also shows you how to keep your digestive tract clean and build up your immune system to prevent further attacks. My frustration is that the conventional medical approach only leaves time, for example, to prescribe 'Canestan' pessaries to a woman who has repeated thrush before her period, without ever attempting to educate her on why this is happening and how to prevent further infections.

Light on a dreary subject

A book on bloated, aching abdomens, swollen sore penises and unpleasant discharges from the vagina cannot exactly be described as light reading, but I trust you will find its pages revealing and optimistic. I also anticipate that you will take heart from the case histories of the people, whose illness has previously defied diagnosis, who have finally, through their own searching, overcome years of physical or psychological problems. It is quite an ascent from being a helpless 'thick-file' patient to being a healthy human being with a good knowledge of how to stay that way.

The good news

As I take up my pencil to start to write this book the words of my old Sister Tutor ring in my ears: 'First reassure the patient'. So I am trying to be an obedient – if somewhat ancient – student nurse when I say that no matter how closely you identify your symptoms with the more severe form of the condition described in this book (systemic candidiasis), and although the list of symptoms looks awesome, do not be alarmed: treatment is effective and you can be well again.

How long will it take

For long-term sufferers I do not pretend that the book offers overnight cures. Several months of treatment might be necessary. Taking a long, hard look at how you are living your life and why you are hurting yourself might also be an important part of the treatment for you. Some people find the physical treatments, such as diet and supplements, relatively easy, but resist change of lifestyle, giving up destructive thought patterns and establishing a relationship with their 'inner child'. I believe that total health depends on the harmony of body, mind and spirit. Loving the inner child (this will be covered later) opens the door to what Jung called 'individuation' – the bringing of the personality and the soul together – and thereby ending the fight which causes tension and renders the body susceptible to illness of all kinds.

Using your recovery time to the full

Tackling any health problem can be a time for personal growth, a time to stop rushing around, a time to make a space in which you can not only understand your needs and make them known to those around you, but also a time when you can lovingly meet those needs. Your first duty is to yourself.

1

The Candida Question

I must also say at the outset, although I am a teacher of self-help and work with complementary medicine, I still have one foot in the other camp and say that self-diagnosis is dangerous and you must describe your symptoms to your doctor before you embark on self-help programmes.

Candida albicans (thrush); why write a book on an organism that is normally present in the gut of every individual soon after birth, a yeast commonly thought to be responsible for little more (except in severely ill people) than infections of the mouth, vagina and irritating skin rashes? The answer is that twentieth-century living – the environment, prescribed drugs (including the pill), street drugs, the ever-increasing consumption of alcohol, junk food, additives, sugar, and the pace of modern living – is slowly changing the human immune system. A healthy gut is an important part of the immune system. It needs to be a balanced ecological system, an environment where there are enough useful bacteria to attack harmful bacteria and keep the growth of fungus (yeasts) at bay, rather like keeping the weeds in the garden under control.

What an overgrowth of candida can do

When candida or other harmful yeasts rule, the sites in the bowel where substances called enzymes live, which are necessary for the breakdown of the food we eat, become blocked. This results in poor digestion, food intolerances, bloating, and altered bowel habits. An overgrowth in the colon can also inhibit the absorption of essential nutrients. That is why so many people on perfectly adequate diets can have vitamin and mineral deficiencies. In addition, the vitamins normally manufactured in the bowel cannot be produced when the colon is in this state, and thus the problem is compounded.

When there is a proliferation of candida it can change from its simple form, which looks like a microscopic fried egg, to a complicated invasive form which grows tentacles which are able to penetrate the bowel wall. This not only allows the toxins (which include alcohol) produced by the candida to circulate, but also gives

5

the organism transport to other parts of the body where infections can arise, resulting in any of the following symptoms.

Physical symptoms

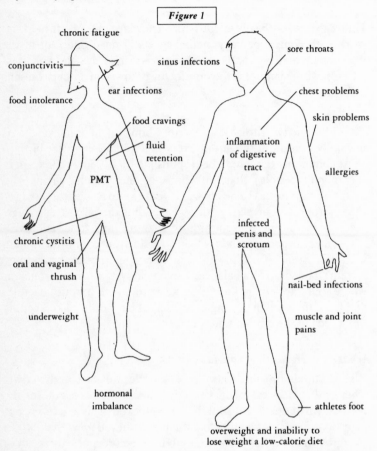

Figure 1

chronic fatigue

conjunctivitis

sinus infections

sore throats

food intolerance

ear infections

chest problems

food cravings

skin problems

fluid retention

inflammation of digestive tract

PMT

allergies

chronic cystitis

infected penis and scrotum

oral and vaginal thrush

underweight

nail-bed infections

muscle and joint pains

hormonal imbalance

athletes foot

overweight and inability to lose weight a low-calorie diet

Brain symptoms

The toxins from the candida can also cause severe psychological symptoms such as agitation, mood swings, anxiety, insomnia and depression.

The medical argument

Because of general lack of awareness on this subject and possibly the diversity of the symptoms, which could be interpreted as hypochondriasis, the long-term sufferer often has endless tests without the condition being diagnosed. If treatment is given, it is often in the form of antibiotics which aggravate the symptoms, or alternatively, the patient is told 'This is only your nerves – why not take a holiday?'

Some doctors believe there is no foundation for the condition chronic candidiasis,[1] others say that the abdominal symptoms may only be the result of fermentation in the gut.[2] Fermentation, as any amateur brewer knows, needs yeast! Two American doctors, O. C. Truss and William Crook, believe that candida can cause widespread problems in the body and have done much to raise 'candida consciousness' both for the medical profession and the sufferer. There are also doctors in this country who work in nutritional medicine (British Society for Nutritional Medicine: see Useful Addresses) who are trying to get the message across. Generally, however, real understanding of the ever-growing fungal problem is in its infancy. It is hoped that the ten-year study on gut fermentation/candida currently being planned at the Middlesex Hospital comes to fruition. When the evidence appears in medical textbooks the situation should be greatly improved.

My experience of working in the community for 15 years leads me to believe that any condition which the average doctor has not met in medical school, in his or her mind does not exist. In saying that, please do not think I am without respect for the medical profession; I have met many doctors who are open and don't let the white coat (and the fear) cloak their own intuitive knowledge, who can let their patients express fully their intuitive feelings about their own bodies before they reach for the prescription pad. Again, I am not anti-drug, but very much against some of the lethal pharmacological cocktails so commonly prescribed in these 'pills-for-all-ills' days. I am also concerned by the endless repeat prescriptions for 'safe' drugs, such as medication for gastric ulcers. I have seen too many prescribed-drug damaged people, and, in this case, many who now face their doctors with chronic conditions, including candidiasis, which have resulted directly from their drug treatment. Not that drugs are the only cause of the candida problem; this will become clearer as you read on.

What is fungus?

The fungi family include moulds, mushrooms, yeasts and rusts.

They are simple plants which lack chlorophyll and are either parasitic, living off live matter, or saprophytic, living off dead matter.

Yeasts are single-cell organisms which reproduce by budding (the formation of a small outgrowth which grows and breaks off) and possess enzymes capable of converting sugar into ethanol (alcohol). This process, called 'fermentation', causes the release of carbon dioxide. In bread-making the dough 'rises' because of this gas. Other products of fermentation are citric acid, oxalic acid, and butyric acid (see page 30). These are formed by certain bacteria.

Fungus is a mass of fine threads from which branches grow upwards. Spores are released from spore cases at the end of each branch. These grow into a new individual and can be carried by the wind.

Fungi are all around us: in our bodies, in the soil and in the air. Some are helpful to us for digestion, baking, brewing and producing antibiotics; others are responsible for diseases in humans, animals and plants.

Is it only candida that causes problems?

No. The fungi which cause infections are too numerous to mention but for the purposes of this book the term fungus will be used except where the yeast *Candida albicans* is known to be the definite culprit. If the body is weakened by an overgrowth of candida in the bowel, other fungi can intrude and the virulence of some of the harmful bacteria can also be increased.

What can I do to cope with fungal infections?

- Clean the colon.
- Stop feeding the fungus – diet.
- Kill the fungus, with drug or non-drug antifungal agents.
- Replace the good bacteria in the gut – probiotics.
- Boost the immune system, with nutritional supplements, and by taking care of general health.

We shall be looking further at each of these later in the book.

Notes

1 'Candidiasis: current misconceptions', *CMAJ*, Vol. 139, October 1988.
2 K. K. Eaton, 'Gut Fermentation: a reappraisal of the old clinical condition with diagnostic tests and management: discussion paper', *Journal of the Royal Society of Medicine*, Vol. 84, November 1991.

2

The Likely Candidates

It has been said that there is an increase in fungal infections in the population generally because of modern living. Predisposing factors which make some people particularly vulnerable are listed below:

- Any debilitating illness which weakens the immune system, such as flu, pneumonia, cancer or AIDS.
  (When the body already has more work than it can cope with, it cannot be vigilant enough to keep harmful organisms in the gut under control. In addition, immunosuppressant drugs, often vital in life-threatening diseases, encourage the body to play host to candida and other fungi. Adequate nutrition and supplements can prevent fungal overgrowth in seriously ill patients and very much improve their prognosis and quality of life.)
- Frequent treatment with antibiotics in the present or past.
- Using the contraceptive pill.
- Taking some prescribed medication (or, more commonly, after withdrawal from); for example: steroids, ulcer drugs, tranquillizers and sleeping pills, long-term antacids.
- Malnutrition: lack of vitamins and minerals, high refined carbohydrate diet, junk foods.
- Stress.
- Endocrine disorders, diabetes.
- Genetic inability to cope with candida or carbohydrate.
- Anaemia.
- After any surgery, particularly abdominal surgery.
- Bowel infections, gastroenteritis.
- Damage to the urinary tract – catheterization.
- Hormonal imbalance: the premenstrual phase, pregnancy, the menopause.
- Multiple pregnancies.
- Ill-treating the immune system: lack of exercise, fresh air, polluted working environment.

- All street drugs.
- Alcohol.
- Lack of hydrochloric acid.
- Infection from sexual partner.
- A history of:
  - repeated bacterial infections
  - hyperactivity as a child
  - allergies
  - swollen painful joints for no apparent cause
  - oral thrush
  - mouth ulcers
  - chronic catarrh
  - erratic vision: spots before eyes
  - vaginal thrush, vulval itching
  - itchy rectum or anus
  - cystitis-like symptoms
  - severe PMT
  - unexplained mild raises in temperature
  - jock itch
  - athlete's foot, ringworm, psoriasis, nail-bed infections (a different organism but often associated with candida), acne
  - craving for sweet or yeast-containing foods
  - being worse after refined carbohydrates, alcohol, cheese, marmite, citrus juice, vitamin B or vitamin C tablets, soft drinks containing citric acid
  - associating abdominal distension, breathing problems or any other symptoms with proximity to some chemicals
  - wind, bloating, cramps, constipation, diarrhoea
  - being weather-sensitive, worse in humid or wet weather
  - being worse in musty or mouldy places
  - irritability, confused thinking, poor memory, being 'spaced out', feeling drunk without alcohol, depression.

Many people say 'but I haven't had thrush or ear problems, etc. for years'. If your body has been coping with an overgrowth of candida for some time it may no longer be responding with acute infection. In effect it has become tolerant to the effects of the organism.

This chapter has given enough details for you to decide whether or not candida could be your problem. It is not an invitation to self-diagnose, but an opportunity for people whose symptoms have been investigated by a doctor to look for other avenues of help. People who have either been told that there is no apparent reason for their problems, or that it is 'just their nerves'.

Brain symptoms

It has been said that in chronic sufferers the body stops reacting with acute symptoms. Persons with 'brain symptoms' may present with vague symptoms of feelings of a permanent hangover (remember, the candida produces alcohol) and of feeling exhausted without being able to pinpoint specific problems. Such people often say 'I feel poisoned and depressed – I have no interest in anything.'

The waste products of the candida can escape from the 'leaky bowel' into the bloodstream and in fact do just that – poison the brain. When the biochemistry of the brain is seriously affected it gives rise to psychological symptoms, but in this instance these symptoms have their foundation in a physical cause. It is therefore useless to treat the brain symptoms of candidiasis, which can range from feelings of hopelessness, irritability, confusion, anxiety and depression to a schizophrenic-like state, with tranquillizers, antidepressants or psychotherapy. Not that psychotherapy isn't useful, since such sufferers can well have life problems because of their condition, but this must be as an adjunct to anti-candida treatment.

How do you know it's not just depression?

It is true that the above symptoms appear in any depressive state and also that many depressed people feel overwhelmingly that there is something physically wrong with them. But where there is any significant history, particularly if there are allergies concerned, and especially where the person has already failed to respond to antidepressants, it is worth trying the anti-candida approach.

Systemic candidiasis

Lisa had been ill for four years. After a period of prolonged stress she developed recurrent thrush, cystitis and severe premenstrual tension. These problems were all new to her and she became increasingly anxious and depressed. Her boyfriend and colleagues began to lose patience with her. She feared her job could be in jeopardy. She had formerly enjoyed her work, but particularly when she was premenstrual, she became very anxious about going to the office because she reacted so explosively to events which she knew would previously have caused her merely to feel mildly irritated. Visits to the doctor resulted in 'Canestan' cream for the thrush, or antibiotics for the cystitis. She was also urged to stop worrying.

Although she was losing weight, her abdomen grew alarmingly. She could not fasten her skirts. This coincided with altered bowel habits: bouts of constipation, then diarrhoea. Even when her stool was loose she felt 'windy' and never felt she had cleared her bowel. This was diagnosed as Irritable Bowel Syndrome which her doctor said was due to nerves. He suggested a high-fibre diet and again to stop worrying.

Two months later when the next set of symptoms arrived, she saw another doctor in the practice. She complained of swelling inside her nose, aching sinuses and a dry cough. She also mentioned she felt ill when she ate certain foods and when she was near some chemicals. The symptoms associated with food intolerance were palpitations, restlessness, depression and nettlerash (hives). The effect of the chemical intolerance was a feeling of being 'spaced out', headaches and inability to concentrate. The smell in her new car and from the photocopier at work seemed particularly to affect her.

She left the surgery with a prescription for a nasal spray and antihistamines. Both helped a little but she was still dissatisfied. She began reading health magazines and books and was delighted when she read an article in a newspaper by a woman who had an identical experience to her own. Armed with information on systemic fungal infections she saw yet another doctor in the practice. To her surprise and delight he agreed this could be the problem and prescribed 'Nystatin'. She put herself onto a strict anti-candida diet and for the first three weeks felt 'rough'. New symptoms developed which she rightly ascribed to 'die off'. The symptoms were slight temperature, feelings of confusion, and muscle and joint pains. As these cleared she made steady progress and said all the symptoms she had suffered for years just seemed to drop away. Friends commented on her appearance: her face regained its normal con-tours (it had been bloated) and was free from the bumps under the skin and dryness that had contributed to her misery over the years.

Lisa's story illustrates the diverse nature of the picture of chronic candidiasis, how seriously the hormone balance can be upset, and also how using 'Nystatin', which should in theory, only work in the digestive tract, can restore immune competence by killing the candida there and allowing the body to cope with infections in other sites. Presumably this happens when toxins from the candida and the undigested particles of protein have stopped leaking from the infected bowel.

Candida and women

It is understandable that there is a higher incidence of candidiasis in women than in men. Oral contraceptives and hormonal influences must be the major reason for this. Candida in the bowel manufactures close on fifty chemicals; some of these are female hormones. The close proximity of the perineum (the area between the anus and the vagina), and also the relatively short length of the urethra (the tube leading to the bladder), could account for women having more acute infections. Nevertheless, men are by no means immune from candidiasis and the numbers of sufferers are increasing. When an overgrowth is established in the bowel they suffer the same digestive problems, allergies, brain symptoms, and so on, as women.

The premenstrual phase and candida

Any hormone disturbance can trigger an acute attack of thrush. Oral contraceptives have been shown to increase the vaginal glucose content by 50 to 80 per cent,[1] thus providing a good food supply for the candida. In the premenstrual phase, during pregnancy and during steroid medication, the delicate acid/alkaline balance of the vaginal secretions is altered. This also encourages fungal growth.

The menopause and candida

During the menopause the vagina can lose its natural lubricant protection and become dry and cracked. This condition is called *atrophic vaginitis* and is caused by a decrease in the oestrogen levels. When the tender mucous membrane of the vagina is torn, candida easily gains entry. Oestrogen creams are often prescribed for this, or a simple lubricant such as KY jelly. There are natural ways of increasing oestrogen levels. Boron, a substance found in vegetables, widely available as a food supplement in health food shops and from nutritional suppliers, has been found to be as effective as hormone replacement therapy. Cold bathing (see page 81) has also been found to raise oestrogen levels.

Thrush

Almost twenty years ago VD clinics reported the incidence of thrush in female patients examined to be as high as 28 per cent.[2] Judging by the alarming increase in prescriptions for vaginal pessaries and creams the figure must be a great deal higher than that now. Repeated thrush infections – which often go hand-in-hand with cystitis (see Chapter 4) – can make life a misery. Acute attacks are characterized by itching and soreness of the vagina and labia with a creamy white or yellow discharge which can have a 'cheesy' odour. Vaginitis caused by *Gardnerella* bacteria produces a greyish frothy discharge which can be mistaken for thrush. If you have an infection which does not respond to anti-candida treatment you could have *Gardnerella* and would need to see your doctor. 'Flagyl' is usually prescribed. Women with *Gardnerella* who are prone to thrush may have a combined infection necessitating both anti-bacterial and anti-fungal treatment. Infection by the parasite *Trichomonas vaginalis* is also sometimes confused with thrush. The symptoms are similar but the discharge is usually darker and the smell stronger. 'Flagyl' is also prescribed for this condition. For non-drug preparations which are effective against fungal, bacterial and parasitic infections see pages 53–7.

An isolated attack of thrush which clears quickly with treatment is of no consequence. The fungus may gain entry because of some slight injury to vaginal tissue, either by vigorous sexual intercourse, a tampon, clothes chafing, or horse riding. Long hot hours sitting whilst travelling, particularly in nylon underwear or tight jeans, can also precipitate an attack. If however you are having regular infections, even if they do clear with Canestan cream, you should be investigating why this is happening. Look at the predisposing factors:

- How stressed are you?
- Is your immune system working well?
- Do you have a healthy diet?
- Is your partner reinfecting you?

Women with a reservoir of candida in the bowel or deep in the vagina are more likely to suffer repeated attacks of thrush, although some women with chronic candidiasis stop reacting with acute attacks. It is common for a chronic candida sufferer to say, 'Oh yes, I had recurrent thrush for years but I don't get it now.' It is important for women who have repeated attacks of thrush to have more than local treatment since it can spread to the reproductive organs and cause pelvic pain.

Treatment

Prescriptions from the doctor would usually be 'Canestan' pessaries or creams. 'Canestan' and 'Daktarin' creams are on free-sale and can be bought in any pharmacy.

Live plain yoghurt is soothing and can clear a mild attack of thrush. Douching twice daily with ten drops of tea tree oil (see pages 62–3) in a pint of warm water or using tea tree cream can be very effective. Tea tree has a mild local anaesthetic effect which is very helpful for itching and soreness. Garlic douches, two crushed cloves in a pint of warm water can also bring relief. 'Cervagyn' vaginal cream, a blend of acidophilus with emollients derived from vegetable oils, helps to maintain normal vaginal flora and penetrates deeply into the vaginal tissue. It has been shown to be a very effective product. It is available in a tube with an applicator from BioCare (see Useful Addresses).

Hygiene

After a bowel movement clean yourself from the vagina towards the anus and if possible wash in cool water. Avoid long, hot baths. Showers are preferable or a warm bath with ten drops of tea tree oil. Juniper and sandalwood oils are also helpful for cystitis – for more information on essential oils, see Further Reading. Empty the bladder and douche with either cool water or one of the suggested solutions after sexual intercourse.

Men can be symptom-free but still carry thrush. It is therefore important for them to pay strict attention to hygiene and to be treated concurrently with their partner.

Clothing

Warm damp conditions encourage thrush, so avoid nylon under-wear, tights and tight jeans. Stockings are the obvious choice but if you prefer tights there are ones without gussets on the market. Since underwear harbours thrush spores wear only white cotton and buy a larger size than usual. They invariably shrink during vigorous laundering. Avoid using wash cloths. To save having to launder a large towel after use, dry the vaginal area with a wash cloth or small towel and disinfect along with underwear. Alternatively, you could dry the area with toilet tissue (preferably unbleached).

When laundering, avoid harsh biological detergents. Old-fashioned boiling in plain water is cheap and safe, or you could scrub the gussets with soap and pour boiling water over them. Treat the gusset of swimwear in this way too, or allow to dry in the sun. Soaking underwear in a solution of tea tree oil and then washing it with the rest of your laundry is another way.

Women, candidiasis and the effects on the brain

The effects on the brain of the chemicals produced by candida and undigested protein have been described. When sufferers present to their doctors with symptoms of lethargy, anxiety, depression and so on, they are often told it's only their nerves, or their symptoms are attributed to their hormones: it's PMT, it's PMT extending over more of the month now that you are past thirty-five, or it's the menopause. Undoubtably part of the story, as we have seen, can be the hormonal influence, but what about the rest, and why do these women *fail* to respond to tranquillizers, antidepressants and treatments for hormonal problems, and recover only when they gain their own knowledge of candidiasis and act on it, or when they see a general practitioner who understands where their symptoms are coming from? Misdiagnosis in women causes frustration, loss of confidence and no doubt in some instances, because of this, psychological problems are superimposed on the existing physio-logical manifestations of altered brain chemistry. Often when a woman feels improvement with anti-candida treatment there will be angry tears: I *knew* it was something in my body that was causing this; why did the doctor not listen to me?

Candida and mothers and babies

Heather Welford is a journalist and writer. She is also a National Childbirth Trust tutor and a breastfeeding counsellor.

Candida can affect the early weeks and months of your baby's life, and bring pain and discomfort to one of motherhood's most pleasurable and rewarding experiences – breastfeeding.

Candida on the nipples, and in the breast itself, can cause

17

soreness, both during feeding and between feeds. It can be bad enough to make even the most dedicated and motivated breastfeeder turn to the bottle in desperation.

Babies, too, can get painful thrush infections on their bottoms and in their genital area. They can also have candida in the mouth, and this may mean it's painful to suck on a breast or bottle.

Thrush and feeding

When a breastfeeding mother complains of soreness, breastfeeding counsellors – mothers trained to help other mothers overcome breastfeeding problems – and professional lactation specialists are usually well aware that thrush could be the reason. But other advisers, including general practitioners, don't always know of the possibility. Mothers are sometimes told to stop feeding, or they're given creams and sprays that have no effect at all on the problem and may make it even worse.

Breastfeeding gives an ideal environment for candida to flourish, especially today in the West, where the breasts might be covered for most of the time with a hot, sweaty, synthetic fabric bra, maybe with a plastic-backed breastpad tucked inside for good measure.

In addition, many new mothers and babies are prescribed antibiotics, often because of a post-natal infection contracted in hospital. Doctors may also prescribe antibiotics as a routine preventive measure to mothers who have had a Caesarean section (13 per cent of deliveries in the UK are now done this way). We've seen on page 10 that antibiotics can make candida conditions more likely.

If either you or your baby has thrush, breastfeeding can mean you pass it between you, backwards and forwards. Bottle-fed babies can get thrush in their mouths, too, as can babies who use a dummy.

Sore bottoms

Nappies are a relatively new invention, and they keep your baby's bottom warm and moist – again, ideal conditions for thrush. The thrush can affect the anus, the buttocks, the genitals and the top of the legs as well.

Symptoms

You may have sore, red, raw or itchy nipples. Sometimes the skin seems to flake away. The nipples are tender between feeds, and it can be very painful when the baby latches on.

However, if you've been sore from the very beginning, then poor positioning (with your baby sucking on the end of your nipple, instead of being well latched on to the breast) is a more likely cause than thrush. Yet you can get thrush on top of soreness caused by poor positioning; and if you're pretty sure your positioning is correct, and you still don't heal, suspect candida.

You may also get intense, stabbing or shooting pains in the breast, most acute when the baby is actually feeding or shortly afterwards. The pains tend to radiate out from the nipple and they may indicate that there is thrush in the breast milk ducts, or in the areas of the breast surrounding the ducts. It is possible to get these pains without any soreness on the nipples.

If your baby is affected by thrush, he or she may have a red, shiny patchy rash on his or her nappy area that doesn't go away with the usual remedies for nappy rash (exposing the bottom to the air, application of nappy rash cream, frequent nappy changes). The effects can be painful, and cause your baby some distress. That's not always the case, however; even quite dramatic-looking symptoms may not produce any soreness.

Oral thrush shows up as whitish deposits in your baby's mouth: on the tongue, the inside of the cheeks and the gums. A few babies show some reluctance to feed and cry when they suck. However, some babies with thrush don't show any symptoms; it is still sensible to assume that if you have it, and you're breastfeeding, then your baby has it too.

Treatment

- Discard all the teats and dummies you're using and buy new ones (sterilize them before use, of course). The same goes for any nipple shields. Shields are sometimes used to protect sore nipples, but they can make the problem worse not better, and they don't help the baby learn to latch on to the breast comfortably. Ask for help in positioning your baby on the breast so you no longer need a shield.

- Wear a cotton bra, and change your breastpads often. Use non-plastic-backed ones.

- See your doctor for anti-fungal medication, and insist on treatment for both you and your baby if you're breastfeeding. Really persistent candida can take a couple of weeks or more to clear, though you should see an improvement in a few days.

- Make sure you pay extra attention to family hygiene, wtih separate flannels and towels for each of you. Check other members of the family for candida, especially your sexual partner.
- If the thrush persists, check your diet (see page 65) and try some of the suggestions in Chapter 7.

Trisha had been feeding baby Joshua for nine weeks, with no problems at all. Then she developed sore nipples. She described them as 'feeling raw'. Feeding was very painful, and her nipples were tender between feeds, too. Her doctor could give no explanation as to why she should develop the soreness after so many weeks of happy feeding, and prescribed some lanolin cream to soothe them. This, if anything, made the problem worse.

By chance, Trisha met a breastfeeding counsellor at a mutual friend's house. The counsellor said the problem could be caused by candida, and this seemed even more likely when Trisha reported a recent bout of vaginal thrush, which had started after a course of antibiotics for an infection.

Trisha's GP was willing to consider this diagnosis, and when Trisha went back he prescribed two separate anti-fungal preparations, one for her and one for Joshua. In a few days. the soreness had gone.

Heather Welford

Men and candida

Men going to the doctor with intestinal candida are more likely to be told they are suffering from diverticulosis or stress. Women are usually given the diagnosis of Irritable Bowel Syndrome, are said to be suffering from the hormone imbalances (the parallel of this in men is lethargy and ill temper) mentioned earlier, or, of course, stress, the 'empty nest syndrome', and so on.

The chronic symptom picture in men is identical to that in women: the same physical symptoms, the same 'neurotic' symptoms. The only differences are obvious biological ones: more alcohol-related candida and more chemical intolerances due to exposure in the workplace. They suffer just as much from digestive problems and food allergies, in fact probably more because it often takes some time to wean them away from a pie and a pint at lunchtime. The case history on page 45 describes the devastation systemic candidiasis can cause in a man's life and that story is by no means unusual.

Acute attacks

Infection around the genitals – 'jock itch' – is common. If the penis is inflamed it is more likely to be a combined bacterial and fungal infection. Thrush manifests in some men as NSU (non-specific urethritis). This needs medical attention since it can lead to a more serious condition called Reiter's syndrome, consisting of arthritis, urethritis, conjunctivitis and sometimes fever and rashes. Boys with candida problems can have severe acne. Men suffer more from athlete's foot than women. If attacks persist after strict hygiene, local treatment, wearing cotton socks, airing shoes and not wearing the same pair every day, then the general health may be low or there could be an overgrowth of candida in the bowel.

Contact dermatitis/candida

Contact dermatitis from buckles on belts, metal on jeans or from washing powders is often complicated by fungal infections and can be very persistent. If your efforts at finding the offending material and using an anti-fungal cream fail, it is advisable to see your doctor.

Avoid synthetic trousers, tight jeans, nylon underwear and Y-fronts (even cotton ones). Boxer shorts allow better circulation of air.

Other causes

Because of raised glucose levels in the blood, diabetic men are prone to fungal infections. The perspiration can often smell 'yeasty'.

Heavy drinking not only feeds candida but also depletes the immune system, disturbs blood glucose levels and prevents the absorption of nutrients which help to control fungal growth. Irritable Bowel Syndrome is common in drinkers or people who have been heavy drinkers in the past. For some reason the frank signs of fungal infections often do not appear until the person has cut down or stopped drinking. It is not uncommon to see recovering alcoholics covered in fungal rashes. They can be anywhere, but more commonly on the trunk and arms, and can persist for months. It could be more than coincidence that psoriasis worsens in drinkers. It is obviously better for drinkers to abstain totally during candida treatment but some are unwilling to do this. Symptoms can improve, however, if they limit their intake and pay more attention to diet and general health, take anti-fungal substances and nutritional supplements.

Notes

1 H. Korte Sneft, *W. Chemotherapy* 28 (Suppl 1), 1982, pp. 13-13.
2 Al Hilton, D. W. Warnock, *British Journal of Obstetrics*, GB1.82, 1975, pp. 922–926.

3
Allergies and Food Intolerance

An allergic reaction is an inflammatory response by the body to a substance to which it is exposed, either by inhalation, ingestion or through contact with the skin. Common allergic responses are seen in asthma, nettlerash, hay fever and eczema. Extreme reaction to one or two foods which have to be avoided for a lifetime can also happen. Symptoms can be severe, sometimes necessitating brief admission to hospital. They include: itching, difficulty in breathing, swelling of the lips, tongue and throat, and nausea. This is a well-recognized medical condition. What is perhaps less well documented is sensitivity or intolerance to several foods.

Food Intolerance

This is also known as masked or hidden allergy. This happens with foods which are eaten regularly; when they are stopped, cravings and other withdrawal symptoms can develop. The diagnosis is not well recognized, possibly because the symptoms can be vague and confused with other conditions, particularly psychological problems; the patient is often dismissed as neurotic. The symptoms look very much like those of candida overgrowth and the two conditions usually co-exist. They are:

- flushing, sweating after meals
- foul taste in mouth, loss of taste
- sore mouth, mouth ulcers
- abnormal thirst
- asthma
- hives (nettlerash)
- inflamed digestive tract
- bloating
- continuous dull abdominal ache
- constipation
- diarrhoea
- flattened stool
- feeling of never having a complete bowel movement
- itching anus

23

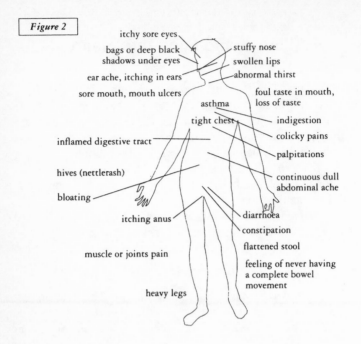

Figure 2

itchy sore eyes
bags or deep black shadows under eyes
ear ache, itching in ears
sore mouth, mouth ulcers
asthma
tight chest
inflamed digestive tract
hives (nettlerash)
bloating
itching anus
muscle or joints pain
heavy legs

stuffy nose
swollen lips
abnormal thirst
foul taste in mouth, loss of taste
indigestion
colicky pains
palpitations
continuous dull abdominal ache
diarrhoea
constipation
flattened stool
feeling of never having a complete bowel movement

- frequency of urine
- urgency of stool
- feeling of the brain being swollen
- irritability, outburst of rage
- feeling of being 'spaced out'
- anxiety or depression after eating certain foods
- chronic fatigue
- hyperactivity

Often these symptoms go on for years, with the sufferer either gaining weight from food cravings, fluid retention, or losing weight because of lack of appetite and anxiety over food. The cry is often, 'All pleasure has gone from eating – just what can I eat?'

Children and food intolerance

Food intolerance in children is becoming increasingly common. Their immune systems cannot cope with modern living: pollution, poor diet and too many antibiotics. They can also be affected by the health of the mother during pregnancy. Children with food

24

intolerances can be pale and listless or pale and hyperactive. Other symptoms are shown in figure 3 below.

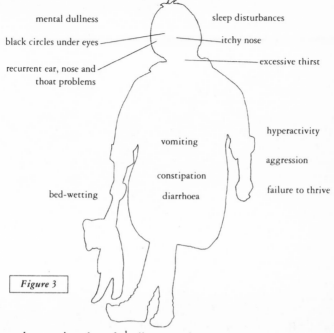

mental dullness

sleep disturbances

black circles under eyes

itchy nose

excessive thirst

recurrent ear, nose and thoat problems

hyperactivity

vomiting

aggression

constipation

bed-wetting

diarrhoea

failure to thrive

Figure 3

In an observational study[1] all cases of a group of children suffering from symptoms of food allergies showed evidence of deficiencies of lactobaccillus and bifidobacterias combined with enterobacteriae (harmful bacteria) overgrowth.

In another study of infants with diarrhoea[2] the main foods implicated were milk, soy and beef.

Soy products

Many adults cannot tolerate soy products, so it is not surprising that it is high on the list of foods causing problems in children. It seems an unnatural diet for infants when you consider they take up to eight ounces at a feed. Perhaps this, and the fact that they have it every day, is one of the reasons for the development of intolerance: the immune system is constantly bombarded and does not have time to recover. Although high in nutrients, beans can be very indigestible. This could be because they contain both starch and protein (see food combining). Doctors can now prescribe soy milk for babies intolerant to cow's milk. Whilst some babies thrive on it, many don't, and both doctor and mother are often slow to suspect the substitute milk because the symptoms do not start immediately, and in fact, after discontinuing the cow's milk, there is often improvement for a time. Here is Joseph's story written by his mother. It is a good example of what has just been discussed.

When Joseph was six months old I stopped breastfeeding and introduced formula cow's milk into his diet. He developed eczema which got progressively worse. After about eight weeks we decided to remove all cow's milk from his diet. As an alternative my GP recommended specially formulated baby soya milk, available on prescription. The eczema improved considerably and I began using other soya products such as yoghurt and custard and all went well, although I did notice Joseph now drank less milk (about half a pint daily). When he was eleven months Joseph caught a stomach bug and had sickness and diarrhoea for several days. We gave him water only and he seemed to recover, although his motions remained very loose with a very acrid, sour smell. After a week or so he vomited violently during the night but seemed fine in himself the rest of the time.

This continued for several weeks: violent vomiting during the night once or twice a week. Continued visits to the doctor were unhelpful; I was constantly told that 'babies were like that' or that it was 'just a bug'.

On his first birthday Joseph was very sick again, but this time he was listless, weak and generally poorly for several days. His abdomen seemed swollen and around his anus was sore. I called out the doctor and was told not to worry.

After a few days on water only Joseph recovered but by now we were anxious; he seemed to be getting thinner and each illness seemed longer and more severe than the last. This pattern continued through December and into January. The bouts of sickness were getting worse and more frequent and Joseph was getting weaker. In between attacks I was giving him as much soya milk as possible in a vain effort to 'build him up'. Finally, in January, he was so poorly – this time his abdomen was very swollen and also his feet were swollen – that I demanded hospital admission. He was there for five days and had blood and stool tests. The doctors found nothing and were baffled by Joseph's condition, which by now had improved although his tummy was still swollen and his rectum remained very red and sore.

I didn't know whether to feel relieved or not. Joseph was discharged and I was told to give him plenty of soya milk and to come back if he became ill again.

By now I was determined to get to the root of the problem and was now convinced that: (a) The original stomach bug back in October had, for some reason, upset Joseph's system so much that he was now unable to tolerate or digest something – but what? Something that had been OK before he got the bug? (b) The solution lay in the elimination of something and the sorting out of Joseph's system.

I was continually searching for answers and by now was so stressed myself I didn't know what to do. It was at this point I decided to seek help from 'alternative' practitioners. I took Joseph to see a homoeopathic doctor and also consulted a nutrition counsellor. Both told me to stop the soya milk and replace it with goat's milk. I diluted it at first and built it up to full strength over a week. Within twenty-four hours we noticed an incredible difference in Joseph. Soya milk had been the culprit all those months. Joseph seemed almost relieved that we had finally solved the problem. He was altogether happier, his skin cleared, his motions were normal and with the help of homoeo-pathic remedies and a careful diet (wheat and yeast-free), he returned to normal. The counsellor asked if Joseph had ever had oral thrush – he had it three times during the early weeks of his life, and I also have a problem with candida.

It is now six months since Joseph was ill. He is thriving, his weight is back to normal and he is a really happy child. His eczema has cleared and he now tolerates cow's milk products. When I look back at the whole experience I think that the worst part of it was that not one of the doctors I saw, even at the hospital, suspected intolerance to soya milk. I have since heard of several similar cases. Why is the medical profession unaware of this problem?

Luke's story

Luke was breastfed until he was five months old and was a contented, cheerful baby. Whilst he was being weaned he became fretful, chesty and had skin rashes. His mother reasoned this was teething. By the time he was two years old he was hyperactive and slept fitfully. His mother thought this was 'the terrible twos' and did not seek help until he started nursery school. The teacher said he was aggressive and difficult to control. When the mother consulted the doctor she was advised to keep him to an additive-free diet. This helped but she still felt that his behaviour was not normal. He could not settle to play with toys or listen to stories the way her two elder children had done, and, although she had no doubt that he was intelligent, she noted that at times he was vague, far away and in her words 'difficult to reach'. He was referred to an allergy unit and was found to be intolerant of sugar and anything in the onion family.

One day he came home from having tea with a friend and 'appeared in a world of his own'. He climbed on the kitchen table and leapt back and forth from the sink unit and working surfaces. This was something he had never done before. He was aggressive when he was restrained. His mother learned later that he had eaten a vegetable burger containing leeks. There had been similar episodes after birthday parties. An exclusion diet greatly improved his symptoms, he was calmer, could concentrate and was now quite happy to play alone with Lego or his train set. He progressed well and only lapsed when he strayed from his diet.

Contributing factors in food intolerances

- Genetic influence.
- Stressed immune system.
- Environmental factors.
- Harmful bacteria, candida overgrowth, parasites in the gut.
- Drugs.
- Inflammation in the gut.
- Damage to gut wall – 'leaky gut'.
- Lack of hydrochloric acid or enzymes.
- Disturbance of pancreatic function.
- Low levels of butyric acid made in the gut.[3]

Food intolerance – the candida connection

Some practitioners believe that overgrowth of candida in the bowel is the major cause of food intolerance. Others believe it is the other way around: stress and environmental factors cause food intolerance and then candida the opportunist takes over when the immune system is too low to fight back. Their answer is to treat the food intolerances first, then the immune system recovers enough to cope with the candida. Their methods are to identify the offending foods or substances by muscle testing (kineseology) and stimulate the body's own defence mechanism by giving homoeopathic doses of the allergens. This is known as desensitization. For a practitioner who uses this approach in your area, see Useful Addresses (Institute of Allergy Therapists).

Allergy testing in the health service

During the past ten years the availability and range of tests for food intolerances in the NHS has increased. Formerly tests were mainly for asthma and hayfever sufferers who were inhaling allergens. Tests now available include:

The skin prick

This is the standard test to see the reaction to common allergens. A drop of the allergen is placed on the skin which is then pricked or scratched. If the patient is sensitive to the drop there is a swelling of the area known as the wheal-and-flare response. This works well for inhaled allergens such as pollens and dust but is unreliable for food intolerances. Sublingual (under the tongue) drops are also used to identify allergens and they are used in diluted concentrations for treatment.

Intradermal injections

These go deeper into the skin than the prick and are more reliable. If the body does not react to the substance it produces a small wheal which soon disappears. A positive reaction increases in size and becomes white and hard.

Neutralization

This treatment is based on finding a dilution of the offending substance which will 'turn off' the allergic reaction by its influence on the immune system. The reason why this works is thought to be unknown but it seems to have close parallels with the homoeopathic principle of like curing like, that is, the correct dilution of whatever the body considers a poison effecting a cure.

Enzyme-potentiated desensitization

This is more likely to be used by doctors outside the health service who work in clinical nutrition. A mixture of food extracts plus an enzyme are applied to a scratch on the skin in a plastic cup. Desensitization is effected in presumably the same way as in the treatments described. One advantage of this method is that it is only needed about once every three months, and less and less as the immune system recovers. Contact Higher Nature (see Useful Addresses) for latest Immuno Test.

Butyric acid for food intolerance

In a healthy gut adequate amounts of this fatty acid are made by the action of bacteria on dietary fibre (fermentation). It appears in large amounts in breast milk. The lining of the bowel has some of the fastest growing cells in the body and butyrates can supply their energy needs and promote natural healing. Low levels of production could precipitate bowel disease in susceptible persons. It has been found to suppress cancer in animal studies and it is thought possible that it could have a role in the prevention of cancer of the bowel.[4] Butyric Acid Complex is available in capsules from Biomed (see Useful Addresses). It should not be used by persons suffering from gastric ulcers or gastritis (inflammation of the stomach). Patients who have been taking from two to four capsules of butyrates at every meal have experienced freedom from many food sensitivities after a period of seven to fourteen days.[5]

Will the doctor be able to help?

The medical evidence for food sensitivities remains controversial because of lack of properly controlled studies; the evidence is mainly anecdotal.[6]

Some people have consulted their doctors for years and have only had endless prescriptions for antacids, preparations for constipation, diarrhoea or colic. These people are often frustrated. Full routine investigations in hospital fail to reveal the cause of their distress, so they just have to live with their symptoms.

Others have been referred by their doctors to the Allergy Unit of their local hospital and have found this helpful to determine which are the offending foods. Others have found the tests in the health service for food allergies unreliable (particularly skin pricks) and have more success following exclusion diets and their own intuition. (CAUTION: Long periods on very restricted diets can lead to vitamin and mineral deficiencies.) If you can afford to see a doctor who specializes in clinical nutrition you will find that not only will the blood or muscle testing used pinpoint your allergies more accurately, but also that you are likely to be given much sounder guidance on diet and supplements.

If you have to rely on your own efforts, do not be too

disappointed because many people have been in the same position and done very well.

How can I find out which food is upsetting me?

The only reliable way is to abstain from foods that you normally eat every day, particularly the ones you feel ill after, and see what happens to your symptoms. You could also try the pulse test, although for some people this may not be necessary because they can feel their heart pounding or missing beats after certain foods. Some doctors say the pulse test is not reliable, reasoning that just because people get anxious and think the food is going to upset them, they experience a rise in pulse rate. This does not explain why they still get reactions when they are not aware of what they are being tested with, as in the 'challenge test' used in hospitals where the patient abstains from certain foods and is given a solution under the tongue to see the reaction. Neither patient nor doctor knows what is in the bottle.

The pulse test

A rise in pulse rate can denote food intolerance. Before using the pulse test, avoid the suspected food for at least five days (some practitioners recommend a month), then take your resting pulse before having a generous helping of the food. Place your palm upwards and press the outer aspect of the wrist with your forefinger, in line with the thumb, and you will feel your pulse.

Count the number of beats in fifteen seconds then multiply by four. This will give the number of beats per minute. If it is raised ten or more beats ten minutes after you have eaten, keep a record of this in a food diary. Take it again after about an hour. Don't rely on memory; keep a record each day of your meals, snacks and drinks and note any symptoms.

Some people don't need to wait ten minutes, or indeed to take their pulse, before their familiar allergic symptoms – heart bumping, headache, wheezing, stuffy nose and so on – descend on them. For some people it only takes two to three minutes. In general the abdominal symptoms take longer to manifest.

If the challenge is too uncomfortable

There are products on the market for symptomatic relief of food intolerance. You might find one in your health food shop or you could send for 'Allergy Switch Off' (£2.85). This is a safe product made from sodium and potassium bicarbonate, and is available from The Sanford Clinic (see Useful Addresses). It is more effective than sodium bicarbonate alone but you could try one teaspoonful of this in a glass of warm water if this is all you have. Some people find eating a large helping of a food they know does not affect them somehow neutralizes the effect.

Keeping cool

All allergies are worse when you are hot. Try splashing the face in cold water, having a cool shower or bath, or resting with an ice pack on the head or abdomen (don't shudder – this can be surprisingly comforting). Ice packs are available at Boots or the Body Shop. A good alternative is an unopened packet of frozen peas. (The peas cannot be returned to the freezer for consumption but only to be used again as an ice pack.) To prevent 'ice-burn', packs should be wrapped in a thin cloth such as a table napkin or tea-towel.

Food rotation

The principle of this diet is rotation and diversification of food. You are most likely to become intolerant of foods you have eaten all your life. Food rotation allows the immune system to recover by not bombarding it with the same allergen every day. Some people react to so many foods that they could not possibly exclude them all because they would become malnourished, so they eat most things, but only once in four days. The body seems to be able to cope with this and many people do well. It is of course tedious, as all these diets are; it would involve eating everything to do with the cow – dairy produce and beef – on one day, and everything connected with sheep – lamb, lamb's liver, ewe's milk yoghurt – on another day, and so on; also a different grain, vegetable and fruit every fourth day. There are many books available which describe food intolerance in detail; see Futher Reading at the end of this book for some suggestions.

Overweight, candida and food intolerances

Sugar and bread craving (the candida constantly crying out for its favourite food) is probably the main cause of overweight in candida sufferers. Altered hormone levels due to the candida could also be a factor. A genetic inability to cope with grains is another possibility. Many overweight sufferers do not make significant progress until they remove all grains from their diet for at least four weeks. No matter how carefully they have dieted, even on one slice of bread per day, they cannot lose weight. Weight loss is often dramatic when they go grain-free (with the possible exception of brown rice and rice cakes). Fluid retention disappears and bloated abdomens improve even if their calorie intake remains the same.

When you eat foods you are intolerant to the cells react by protecting themselves with extra fluid. This can dramatically increase weight. The addiction/allergy connection is very close so you may crave the very foods which are causing your weight problem.

Some people find it difficult to lose weight because they do not eat enough protein to boost their metabolism and keep their blood-sugar levels stable. This also makes them lethargic and so their problem is compounded by lack of exercise. Vegetarians are often in this group. Overweight people are often low in essential vitamins and minerals and have the toxic colon problem.

Underweight and candida

If you are underweight, and particularly if your appetite is poor, consult your doctor or a nutritionist before embarking on an anti-candida diet. If your appetite is good and you can eat much larger helpings of the allowed foods and if the weight loss does not continue (you could expect some at first) then you could see how you fare. Underweight people would do well to investigate the desensitization approach (page 29) which only calls for a reduction in sugar and salt.

Chemical intolerance

Substances which cause the gut to swell and give rise to other symptoms of intolerance don't always gain access to the body through the mouth, but can be inhaled or absorbed through the skin. Be more aware of the chemicals you are spraying on your head, under your arms, up your nose and on your skin. Use simple non-perfumed toilet preparations and don't buy aerosol cans. Anti-perspirants stop natural detoxification through the skin. Use a simple deodorant. Boots have one in their men's range and Vichy also make one which is widely available. Most essential oils are antiseptic and tea tree (see page 62–3) is available as a deodorant stick. Some oils come in a carrier oil such as jojoba and can be used as perfume. They smell wonderful and you are much less likely to be affected by them.

Chemicals in the home and garden

It is time also to throw out all the household cleaning agents and get back to simple soaps (non-biological washing powders) and old-fashioned wax furniture polish instead of spray cans. There is a whole range of ecological domestic cleaning products; the washing-up liquid has been particularly helpful for many people. If you cannot find a safe product make sure you immerse the nozzle of your container so that you don't inhale the droplets, and also rinse the dishes very carefully. There was research some years ago which confirmed that traces of washing-up liquid can irritate the bowel lining. A tight chest whilst washing up is also very common in people with chemical allergies. A simple product called 'Chemico', a pink paste made from powdered rock which has been manufactured in Britain for about seventy years, is a gentle and safe scouring agent. It cleans everything: sinks, cookers, floors, even windows. You might not find it in the supermarket but a hardware store will order it for you. Avoid garden chemicals as much as possible. Frequent hoeing is safer than using noxious weedkillers and washing-up liquid is quite effective for aphids (unfortunately some plants do not like the ecological products). If you have to paint or use wood preservatives, make sure your working space is well ventilated and that you take frequent breaks.

Travelling

Inhalation of the brake fluid on trains causes swollen eyes, headaches and abdominal symptoms in some chemically allergic people. Travelling by car can also be a problem. Keep the windows closed and if possible fit a car ionizer (see page 84); they are inexpensive and well worth the effort. Make frequent stops to escape from fumes. Chemical inhalants from plastics, adhesives and flooring in shopping areas can also cause symptoms in some people. Printer's ink, tobacco smoke, gas, oil, factory fumes, formaldehyde (air fresheners), chipboard furniture, synthetic carpets – although the fumes from these do decrease with time – are all implicated, in addition to the well-known allergens in nature such as pollens, dust mites and so on.

A toxic colon

In time, when you have cleansed your colon and restored the balance of the good and bad bacteria, when you have adequate production of enzymes and your dietary intake and internal production of vitamins is correct, your food intolerance should greatly improve or disappear. Colon cleansing is the first step on the road to recovery.

A toxic colon is not only a major factor in the development of food intolerances and chronic vague ill-health, but it can also cause degenerative disease such as arthritis and cancer. You cannot expect to be well if the main organ responsible for ridding the body of toxic waste is underfunctioning. When the colon is irritated by diet, stress, drugs, chemicals, and so on, it tries to protect itself by producing more mucous; this can bind with the sludge from refined foods, such as white flour, and build up on the wall of the bowel and narrow the lumen. This layer of gluey hardened faeces can weigh several pounds and is a good place for harmful organisms to breed. How this layer prevents the production of enzymes and vitamins, and how it hinders absorption has already been mentioned. Do not think because you have regular bowel movements or even diarrhoea that you have escaped this problem. The stool can pass daily through a dirty colon and leave the accumulated residue on the walls behind. There is no need to get panicky about the amount of weighty garbage you might be carrying around with you: there is a great deal you can do about it.

How this toxic layer can affect the body

The local effects of this poisonous residue are irritation and inflammation; the general effects include diarrhoea, constipation, fatigue, headaches, dull eyes, poor skin, spots, aching muscles, joint pains and depression. The poisons circulate via the blood through the lymphatic system to all parts of the body. Healthy lymphatic fluid should serve to nourish cells not fed by blood vessels. The lymphatic fluid also kills off harmful organisms and carries away the refuse. If the body has to pump around excessive toxic waste long term it is not surprising that it sometimes has to give up and the disease process takes over. It is understandable that there are more and more people referred to hospitals for Irritable Bowel Syndrome, colitis (inflammation of the colon), Crohn's disease (inflammation of the small intestine), colon cancer and diverticulitis.

When the muscles of the colon wall lose tone this results in ballooning or the formation of pouches called diverticula, leading to a condition known as *diverticulosis*. The food trapped in these pockets makes a wonderful breeding ground for bacteria. The result can be diverticulitis, an infection where there is often a fever and acute abdominal pain. This condition needs medical help.

The two diagnoses of diverticula disease and Irritable Bowel Syndrome are often interchangeable. Men are more likely to be told they have diverticula problems; women that they have Irritable Bowel Syndrome. I have covered how to help inflammation of the bowel and the effect of high and low levels of hydrochloric acid in the new edition of my book *The Irritable Bowel Syndrome and Diverticulosis*.

Cleansing the colon

The benefits of colon cleansing are manifold, not only in terms of health but also with regard to appearance: the skin looks vibrant; cellulite, water retention and blemishes disappear; and the whites of the eyes regain a youthful clearness. How quickly you want to clean out is your choice. Some people are so tired of being below par they are willing to endure the effects of rapid cleansing. This does not happen to everyone but it is as well for you to know you could experience migraine, blinding headaches, nausea or flu, aches and pains, fever, exhaustion, and nervous symptoms such as anxiety, panic attacks, irritability, weepiness or even quite profound depression. The worst of this would be over in approximately five days. You might decide to take the process gradually. Changing to a clean diet over a period of several weeks is described in my book on the Irritable Bowel Syndrome. If you also want to lose weight two books on clean eating with a common-sense approach are *The Wright Diet* by Celia Wright and *Fit for Life* by Harvey and Marilyn Diamond.

Cleansing the Colon by Brian Wright (available from New Nutrition – see Useful Addresses) is an excellent booklet which describes how you can achieve a complete colon cleanse by diet, natural supplements and herbs.

If you cannot afford books or supplements, a diet of 50 per cent raw food and taking a teaspoonful of linseed (a bag from the health food shop will last months for a cost of about £2) or taking two level teaspoonsful of Isogel, an old-fashioned inexpensive bulking agent available from Boots and most chemists, would be a good start. You can chew the linseed to release the nutrients. Isogel is easy to swallow if you mix it with yoghurt. Water is essential to clean anything. Aim for two litres per day whilst you are cleansing the colon unless this conflicts with advice from your doctor. At least a half a pint, preferably hot, before breakfast gets the day off to a good start. Some people say that they can't do that because they retain fluid, but some practitioners believe that the body responds with fluid retention when it does not get enough fluid; it tries to hang on to its ration.

How long does it take to clean the colon?

It is unlikely that you will have a pristine inside within a couple of weeks; it could take months. You will know when things are happening: your skin and eyes will look clearer, your digestion will improve, you will have more energy and niggling aches and pains which have been around for years will disappear. You could feel mentally better, too, less jumpy and clearer headed.

Colonic irrigation

Most people think of this as some nightmare experience. It is far from this and a very quick efficient way to loosen the impacted faeces and wash away toxins. It also obviates many of the unpleasant symptoms of detoxification. A sterile tube is inserted into the rectum and filtered water washes around the colon. It leaves via an evacuation tube, taking with it the accumulated debris and mucus of years. If you want to find a practitioner in your area write to the Colonic International Association (see Useful Addresses).

Can vitamins help?

A good intake of the B vitamins is essential. Niacin, Vitamin B^3, is particularly helpful. It has been shown not only to prevent the development of allergies but also to help cramps, and sugar or alcohol craving. It helps detoxification through stimulating the circulation. It has also been found to help nervous symptoms since it closely resembles a group of drugs called the benzodiazepines (Valium, Ativan, etc.). Niacin can produce a harmless flushing or pricking of the skin which disappears in less than an hour. Nicotinamide is a form of B^3 which does not cause flushing. There was a fashion some years ago to give large doses of this vitamin for detoxification, but it was found that patients on sustained medium or high doses sometimes became depressed. This is not surprising since it has been called 'Nature's Valium'. Valium, or any substance which produces over-sedation, can have this effect. The B vitamins are synergistic, that is, they depend on each other for absorption (vitamin B^3 needs vitamin B^6) so it is not recommended that you take any of them in isolation without expert guidance. It is also vital that you choose yeast-free preparations. Some people with bowel problems find even the purest non-allergenic brands give them problems. If this happens to you, cut down the recommended dose and build up gradually or take them two to three times weekly. More about supplements on pages 72–7.

Notes

1 Melvyn R. Werbach MD, *Nutritional Influences on Illness* (Thorsons 1987), p. 27.
2 H. R. Jenkins, et al., 'Food Allergy: the major cause of infantile colitis', *Ann Allergy*, Vol. 153, October 1984.
3 T. Neesby, 'Butyric Acid Complexes: a new approach to food intolerances', *Biomed Newsletter*, Vol. 1, No. 2, February 1990.
4 John H. Cummings, 'Short-Chain Fatty Acids in the Human Colon', *Gut*, Vol. 22, 1981, pp. 763–79.
5 ibid.
6 R. Podell, 'Food Allergy: A mainstream perspective', *Clinical Ecology* 3 (2), 1985, pp. 79–84; Kuvaeval, et al., 'The Microecology of Food Allergy', *Nahrung*, No. 28, 1984, pp. 689–93.

4

Other Fungal Conditions

Cystitis

It is likely that candida can invade the bladder wall in the same way that it attacks the lining of the bowel or the vagina. I have seen hundreds of people here and abroad whose symptoms have failed to respond to antibiotics and whose urine analysis proved negative. Their symptoms *did* however respond finally to anti-fungal medication or to self-help anti-candida methods.

Fungal cystitis

In the main, the symptoms of these people were different from the 'ordinary cystitis' (bacterial) sufferer, those who had isolated attacks causing pain, or burning on passing urine, which had an unpleasant smell and often contained pus or blood. Urgency and frequency are also features of bacterial cystitis. This symptom picture usually responds quite quickly to antibiotics, by contrast to fungal cystitis which does not.

In fungal cystitis the symptoms tend to be less dramatic, more of a background discomfort in the bladder and the urethra which is made worse by drinking citrus juices, alcohol, strong coffee, some soft drinks, and also by yeasty, sugary foods and some vitamin supplements, particularly vitamins C and B complex. It is true that a bladder inflamed by bacteria or viruses would also object to acid drinks, but it is unlikely that normal cystitis sufferers would be affected by eating bread or other foods normally included in their diet.

An important point to remember is that urine specimens sent to microbiology departments are not tested for fungus without a special request. A typical general hospital might expect between 1 and 5 per cent of all urine specimens received for culture to contain yeasts.[1] It is imagined that a large proportion of these specimens would be from patients with indwelling catheters or those who were hospitalized for some serious condition requiring large doses of antibiotics. Few will have come from GPs looking for fungal cystitis in their patients: If you identify your symptoms with those of fungal cystitis it would be wise to ask your doctor if a fungal test could be included in the investigations.

Fungal cystitis can be the only symptom, although it is more commonly seen in people who have fungal infections in other sites, for example, in the gut, vagina (thrush) or nail beds. An irritated bladder can also be a feature of food intolerance.

Proprietary medicines for cystitis

These can bring temporary relief to an inflamed bladder but should not be used for long periods. They work by making the urine alkaline and ease the inflammation in much the same way as an antacid soothes an irritated gastric lining. In both cases it is unwise to use these preparations for prolonged periods because they upset the delicate acid–alkaline balance of the body and lead you into further troubles.

In the case of fungal cystitis it may make you feel more comfortable, but since candida thrives in an alkaline medium it could eventually compound your problem. Some preparations contain citric acid.

Natural remedies for cystitis

Women are more prone to cystitis than men because they have a shorter urethra (tube leading from the bladder) and it is therefore easier for harmful organisms from the bowel to ascend into the bladder. In the article 'Urinary Tract Infection and the Potential for a Natural Prophylactic Treatment'[2] the effect of cranberry juice on urinary tract infections was discussed. There has been evidence for about thirty- five years that it can help to prevent infections. It works by preventing harmful bacteria, particularly *E.coli*, from attaching to the lining of the bladder:

There seems to be little doubt that cranberry juice can be extremely valuable in the prophylaxis [prevention] of urinary tract infections, especially for patients with recurrence. It is probable that the relief of acute infection will always lie in the domain of antibiotics, but as well as other side effects, they do diminish the host's own defences against the recurrence of the disease. Overall, urinary tract infections is such a major problem, notably of female health, that any effective addition to the armoury of the practitioner would be very welcome. One advantage of cranberry juice, is that it cannot possibly do any harm – only good.

Cranberry juice is very popular in America. It can be found in some delicatessens and supermarkets here, or try the off-licence store where it is often stocked as a mixer for vodka. Cranberry juice preparations combined with acidophilus are available from Bio-Care (see Useful Addresses).

Homoeopathy, herbs and essential oils are also used for the relief of cystitis.

At the slightest sign of discomfort in the bladder or urethra drink as much water (preferably bottled) as you can and take warm baths. Sometimes a hot-water bottle on the lower back or abdomen helps.

Even if there is no bacterial or fungal infection in the bladder it can become irritated by eating or drinking something you are intolerant to.

For more on the management of cystitis see Further Reading at the back of this book.

Candida and ME (Myalgic Encephalomyelitis)

ME is a chronic illness thought to be viral in origin which depresses the immune system, and because of this other opportunist viruses, bacteria or fungi step in and produce a bewildering, debilitating illness. The central nervous system can also be affected causing transient paralysis, speech and eating problems and also loss of balance. ME is characterized by bouts of extreme tiredness in the muscles and brain which are not alleviated by rest. This understandably gives rise to feelings of hopelessness and depression. It can start with an illness like glandular fever or flu. Sometimes it is so severe people have to give up work for a time.

Sufferers from this condition have been classed as malingerers or hypochondriacs for decades, and many have been very harshly treated by their medical practitioners. ME was first recorded about fifty years ago, but it has only been in the past few years that there has been a sharing of information amongst sufferers and doctors. It is often mistaken for nervous illness because the symptoms include anxiety, depression and lethargy, and many patients have been labelled hysterics.

Research is being carried out at St Mary's Hospital, London, and elsewhere, but as yet there are few answers in conventional medicine, except where nutritional therapy has been combined with antidepressant medication, particularly the drug amitriptyline. Overall, however, the best results have been reported with the

41

approach of clinical nutritionists who treat nutritional deficiencies (ME sufferers are often found to be low in magnesium), candida and food intolerances.

Treatment

Because the immune system is so low in ME sufferers, yeast-related problems and allergies are very common. Full recovery cannot take place without these conditions being treated.

Other important aspects of treatment are rest, a healthy diet, nutritional supplements (during severe illness or times of stress the body demands greatly increased supplies of essential minerals and vitamins), fresh air, daylight, and keeping the bowel as clean as possible by preventing constipation and restoring the normal balance to the gut bacteria. Any therapy which promotes relaxation and natural healing is also recommended. Tranquillizers rarely help this condition; they merely add more poisons to a body already struggling hard to excrete the poisons caused by the virus. Sometimes a night-time dose of a sedative antidepressant is helpful where insomnia is severe and where normal sleep–wake cycles are trying to be established.

Sufferers need to be believed, reassured that they will recover in time, and to have the nature of the illness fully explained to them. GPs in the London area are able to refer patients to the Homoeopathic Hospital.

For further information about ME see Useful Addresses and Further Reading at the back of the book.

Fungal skin problems

The point to remember about skin problems is that they start on the inside. Localized infections are a sign that the immune system is not as healthy as it could be, so no matter how many times skin problems clear up with creams and so on, they will recur if the body's defences are not kept in good working order. (More about this on pages 46–9.)

Candida is not responsible for all fungal skin problems; more than one parasitic yeast may invade the body when the immune system is low. For example, nail-bed and scalp ringworm are due to dermatophyte fungi (tinea) and whilst they are often seen in people with chronic candida problems they need different systemic and topical treatment. See your doctor if you have candida-like symptoms or skin or nail-bed infections which don't clear up with anti-candida measures (see anti-fungal drugs, page 50).

Neither are all fungal skin problems as dramatic as the ones mentioned in the case histories; nevertheless, some can be distressing, particularly if they are on the face. They usually take the form of a scaly red rash at the sides of the nose and between the eyebrows. If the rash is severe it can extend across the cheeks and can have the appearance of sunburn. The hands can also become very dry. Very often the flare-ups of the skin problems are associated with stress and it is difficult to say how much is fungal in origin and how much can be attributed to candida in the gut causing vitamin deficiencies. It is probably both. During stressful times not only does the immune system have to work harder to keep the candida under control but also the need for some vitamins, particularly the B vitamins, is greatly increased. This is why anti-fungal treatment plus vitamins is much more effective than either treatment alone.

Athlete's foot

This is characterized by itching and redness between the toes. The skin can be flaked, cracked or moist. Footbaths with tea tree oil, the application of neat tea tree oil or proprietary creams plus strict foot hygiene are effective (see page 50).

Nail-bed infections

These can be very stubborn and take several months to clear. Topical application alone is not usually enough. Internal treatment plus regular application of neat tea tree oil or an anti-fungal cream (not 'Nystatin') is necessary (see page 50).

Acne

This disfiguring condition is caused by the hormonal influence on the sebaceous glands. It produces blackheads and pustules on the face, neck and shoulders. It occurs mainly in adolescence but can occur later in life when drugs alter hormone levels. Persons who have had long-term antibiotics for acne in their youth often suffer severe candida problems later in life. It has been said that overproduction of hormones encourages fungal growth and it has been noticed that people having treatment for candidiasis often lose all trace of acne. Acne sufferers are often found to be zinc deficient.

Psoriasis

This is a chronic distressing skin condition characterized by raised, red, scaly lesions. Some scientists believe it to be genetic in origin, others favour hormonal influences, raised cholesterol levels, allergic reactions to food or drugs, whilst others see stress as a major factor with the condition appearing up to two years after a traumatic event. Medical science admits that existing treatments lack efficacy and that some of the drugs used have adverse effects.[3] Nutritional therapists have long associated this condition with a depressed immune system and/or candida. Sufferers are often found to have a marked zinc deficiency.[4] Some American doctors have seen the candida/psoriasis connection for some time. Professor E. William Rosenburg, dermatologist of the University of Tennessee College of Medicine in Memphis, claims a 75 per cent success rate within four months on anti-fungal drugs and sugar/refined carbohydrate/yeast-free diet. Nutritionists recommend a diet high in raw vegetables, fruit and oily fish such as herring and mackerel. A study in America[5] attributed the low level of psoriasis amongst Eskimos to high levels of omega fatty acids found in their mainly fish diet. Herbal remedies and homoeopathy can also be helpful in this condition.

Notes

1 *The Lancet*, 29 October, 1988.
2 *Biomed Newsletter*, Vol. 2, No. 8, 1991.
3 *The Lancet*, 31 August, 1991.
4 *British Journal of Dermatology*, Vol. 123, 1990, pp. 319–323.
5 Geraldine Mccarthy, Medical College of Wisconsin, *The Lancet*,, 28 September, 1991.

5

Case Histories

More serious health problems due to fungal infections are discussed elsewhere in the book. This section highlights the fact that what could be considered minor problems in a medical sense can still cause a great deal of distress and impair the quality of life. The persistent nature of some of these problems and their tendency to recur, often year after year, can lead to a feeling of hopelessness and helplessness.

Swollen sore genitals

A 22-year-old male student described his life as complete misery when he came for help. His penis was so swollen and sore he found walking and even sitting in lectures difficult. In his room he wore only a long T-shirt and outdoors a loose tracksuit. It was impossible to wear jeans, his normal attire. He was also anxious, frustrated and depressed. He had no social life and was very worried about the future.

He had been seeing his doctor for several months and had initially been given antibiotics, and later anti-fungal drugs and cortisone cream. The anti-fungal treatment helped but within a few days of stopping treatment the symptoms returned. He was finally sent to see a consultant at a 'Special Unit' (Department for Sexually Transmitted Disease) and was told he had both bacterial and fungal infections. He was given antibiotics and anti-fungal medication which were more effective than the anti-fungal treatment alone; but, again, once treatment stopped the symptoms returned.

It wasn't until he rang a candida counsellor, who asked about diet and food cravings, that he realized how much he craved cheese and marmite sandwiches and his daily pint of beer. He said he had reasoned that he ate the sandwiches, which were the mainstay of his diet, because they were convenient and economical, but on reflection he said if he ate out he always had one when he returned – the candida screaming for its favourite diet!

Because it was the least expensive he chose the garlic method (see page 53) and made a half-hearted attempt at the candida diet.

Two weeks later his condition had improved but he felt he would have to be stricter about the diet and take some of the suggested supplement. He bought acidophilus and yeast-free mineral and vitamin supplements.

Four weeks later he rang to say he was doing very well unless he reverted to his old habits.

Abdominal symptoms plus recurrent ear infection

A 39-year-old female had successfully withdrawn from tranquillizers after taking them for ten years. Three months after withdrawal she complained of a bloated abdomen, a constant feeling of immanent cystitis and an ear infection. The ear discharged a watery fluid which dried into a crystalline deposit on her skin nearly to her chin. The skin became inflamed and had almost the appearance of a burn.

She was prescribed three different courses of antibiotics without any effect, before a swab was sent to the laboratory. The result confirmed she had a fungal infection. She was given antifungal ear drops and cream for her skin. The ear symptoms needed prolonged treatment but eventually cleared up. Her abdominal symptoms and urinary symptoms persisted until she went on to the anti-candida diet.

Skin problems: pityriasis rosacea

Elizabeth had a history of being given antibiotics for ear infections as a child, and as an adult for a kidney infection. For several years after the kidney infection she had feelings of impending cystitis, often associated with stress or eating certain foods.

After a particularly stressful period she noticed a slight dry rash. It worsened over a period of ten days, until it separated into round red patches about the size of decimal halfpennies. It looked like cigarette burns and appeared on the trunk only, not on the limbs at all and not on the face. Itching was a problem especially when she was hot.

The doctor diagnosed *pityriasis rosacea* and said it was caused by an airborne virus which she could have picked up on a bus, and there was no cure; it would clear up of its own accord within about three months. Elizabeth was horrified at the thought of having such a disfiguring, uncomfortable rash for so long and also realized it would prevent her from swimming or taking exercise which would make her hot.

The name was the clue to the whole business. After her visit to the doctor she remembered her cousin had been diagnosed as having the same condition but her doctor had ascribed it to a fungal infection. She bought a book on candida and started on the anti-candida diet immediately. She was very strict about sugar (even fruit), bread and cheese and not quite so strict with wine and diet Coke. Vegetables, fish, lamb and free-range, corn-fed eggs were the mainstay of her diet. Other red meats and battery eggs were avoided because antibiotics are included in the feed.

Essential oils of lavender and tea tree, three drops of each, were used in the bath daily and two drops of each oil were mixed with one dessertspoonful of olive oil and applied to the rash twice daily. This was very helpful for the itching. She also had a sun bed every three or four days.

A telephone counselling session with a nutritionist from New Nutrition (see page 97) resulted in her starting supplements a few days later. These included caprylic acid, superdophillus, and herbal tablets and psyllium husks as part of the bowel cleansing programme. She also drank the Pau d'Arco[1] anti-fungal herbal tea. For the first week or so after starting the diet, the rash actually got worse. After about ten days there was slight improvement, which was definite a few days later. After that she said she could see it clearing before her eyes; it seemed to retreat inwards, being most stubborn in the warmer places, around the armpits and stomach.

Three weeks after her first visit to the doctor she went back to show him the results. Her skin was almost perfect in a fraction of the time he had told her. He was astonished but did not show any interest in how she had cured herself. He was pleased, but just seemed to think it was a bit of unusual good luck.

Elizabeth's story illustrates how attacking fungal skin infections from inside and outside can achieve rapid results. Fungal skin problems need not be as dramatic as this; they can come and go, depending on how stressed you are or what you are eating.

47

Tender cracked finger tips

Mavis had suffered from sore fingers for years. When they were at their worst the tips would crack and bleed. She had tried creams from the doctor and wearing gloves for housework but these measures did not help. She was elderly and on a low income, so she was advised to try simple things first, such as cutting down on sugar and tea and eliminating wheat altogether, substituting Ryvita for bread. She was encouraged to eat more vegetables and take one multimineral and one multivitamin tablet daily (both yeast-free). Three days after giving up bread she saw improvement and after a week her fingers had completely healed. For three weeks she was delighted: she could knit, sew and do her housework without any problems. She then decided to try bread again to see what would happen – she had half a slice of bread; the following day her fingers were inflamed and sore. She stayed wheat-free for three months, then found she could eat a scone or bread two to three times a week without problems.

It could be said that Mavis' sore fingers were due to a wheat allergy and not fungal infection. Experience has shown, however, that candida and allergy very often go together, and in this instance it did not matter. The simple suggestions cleared up a long-standing painful condition. She rightly said that skin problems often seem to be a neglected area of medicine. Since they are not life-threatening and people are usually still mobile, they are often left to get on with them.

Severe itching of the scrotum and groin

It can be seen from John's story that fungal problems can arise in people who are perfectly healthy when they include something in their diet which causes the candida in the bowel to multiply.

John telephoned to say he had an unbearably itchy rash around his anus, scrotum and up into his groin. He was losing sleep, becoming irritable and finding it impossible to sit still in meetings. His work was suffering because of poor concentration. Sitting in cold water was the only way he could ease the itching. The creams he had been given by the doctor worked to some extent but the effect did not last.

He was questioned on his diet and lifestyle and both of these seemed healthy: adequate exercise, lots of vegetables, salads, fruit and fish, a non-smoker who drank moderately at weekends only. All was revealed when he was asked about stress at work. He replied that things had been a bit hectic at work since Christmas but he was taking brewer's yeast tablets for extra B vitamins. He said his colleague had recommended them. When asked if he associated the onset of his symptoms with taking the tablets he replied it had not occurred to him. He thought they were an old-fashioned, healthy addition to the diet and even if they did not do very much at least they could not do any harm.

On reflection he saw the connection: he started the tablets the week before a conference and slight itching had started the following week. It gradually became more severe and had continued to date. All he did to cure himself was to stop the tablets and drink lots of water. Two days later he rang to say he was much improved; a week later his skin was back to normal.

Chemical intolerance

Adrian had been unable to work for three months. His diagnosis was ME(?) depression(?). His bowel problems started whilst he was travelling in India. He had been home a year and was not having such trouble with his bowel but seemed to be allergic to 'everything in sight'. Paint, cigarette smoke, or even pottering in the garden shed or in the garden on a 'mouldy' day could make him feel weak and exhausted for several days. He began to feel like a prisoner; his wife said he was neurotic and his self-esteem was at an all-time low.

Information from an ME self-help group gave him hope. He saw a clinical nutritionist privately and after six months' anti-fungal, nutritional therapy he felt back to his former self.

Notes

1 Pau d'Arco is an anti-fungal tea also known as Taheebo, Lapacho, and Upe Roxo. It is made from the unsprayed bark (the tree is unharmed by the harvest) of the Inca Bow Tree. The Inca Indians made bows from these trees and drank the tea from the bark. They thought its effects were miraculous. It is bio-chemically complex and contains Lapachol.

6
Looking for Answers

Anti-fungal drugs

Anti-fungal drugs are effective but some are not without their problems.

- *Diflucan* (fluconazole) is increasingly being used for candida. For systemic candidiasis doctors usually give 50 mg a day for two weeks, followed by a single 150 mg dose weekly for several weeks. 150 mg capsules are now on 'free sale'. A single capsule will usually clear thrush. Check with your pharmacist for possible interactions if you are taking other drugs. Also ask about other contraindications.
  Note: People often consult nutritionists for natural anti-fungal substances after being treated with Diflucan, not only because of toxic reactions but also because they experience a very rapid return of the candida as soon as the drug is discontinued.
- *Amphotericin* (Fungilin) is used for systemic fungal infections and is effective against most fungi and yeasts. It is however toxic and side-effects are common. They include digestive upsets, headaches and joint pains.
- *Griseofulvin* is well absorbed from the gut and is often used when infections of the skin, scalp and nails have failed to respond to creams and lotions. The side-effects are headache, digestive upsets and sensitivity to light.
- *The imidozole group* – clotrimazole, econazole, ketonconzole and miconazole – are active against a wide range of fungi and yeasts. Oral use, except for miconazole which is used for mouth and intestinal infections because of the risk of liver damage, is normally only used in severe resistant infections. The drugs in this group are used widely in pessaries, creams, sprays and powders. Many are available on free sale in pharmacies. They include 'Canestan' (clotrimazole) and 'Daktarin' (miconazole).
- *'Nystatin'* is an older drug which is not absorbed from the gut. This makes it less effective for systemic candidiasis. It is used for intestinal, vaginal and skin infections due to candida. In common with amphotericin it is ineffective against tinea (ringworm). The side-effects can be less than with some of the other anti-fungal drugs although what is known as the Herxheimer reaction or

dieback can occur. As the drug kills the yeast cells they burst and release toxins into the bloodstream. If this is done too rapidly the effect can be similar to flu: raised temperature, headaches, nausea, aches and pains. The problem can be minimized by gradually building up to the recommended dose or by reducing the amount of candida in the bowel by careful dieting for about a month before drug treatment. The tablets available on the NHS do not dissolve until they reach the large bowel. They would therefore miss infection anywhere else in the digestive tract. This could be helped by crushing them and putting them in water.

When 'Nystatin' powder is used it is much easier to graduate the dose and it also treats the whole of the digestive tract. If your doctor is willing to prescribe this the supplier could be found through the British Society for Nutritional Medicine (see Useful Addresses). He or she may be happier to prescribe this rather than one of the newer non-drug anti-fungals because it has been used by the health service for so long.

Prescribed drugs which favour the growth of candida
* *Antibiotics*
Antibiotics encourage candida overgrowth because they are not selective and destroy useful and harmful bacteria simultaneously.
* *The pill*
Disturbances in hormone levels could be one reason why the pill encourages candida; another could be that in women who take the pill the prevalence of abnormal glucose (sugar) tolerance is increased from approximately 4 to 35 per cent.[1] If the blood glucose levels are raised (hyperglycaemia) there is more food for the candida, as in diabetes.
* *Corticosteroids*
Again hormone levels will be disturbed, and also these drugs have a much greater influence than other groups of drugs upon glucose tolerance.[2] Drugs like 'Prednisone', steroid asthma inhalers and even creams in large doses can have this effect.
* *Other drugs which effect raised glucose levels*
These include diuretics, beta blockers, Epanutin[3], Cimetidine, Ranitidine (for gastric ulcers). These drugs are extremely useful for the treatment of gastric ulceration and have saved countless numbers of people from surgery. Unfortunately because they are considered safe they are abused in general practice. They are often prescribed at the slightest sign of gastric disturbance

(without ever a thought to the patient's eating habits or lifestyle) and repeat prescriptions are issued for years without any reassessment of the patient's condition.

• *Laxatives*

Overuse of strong laxatives prevents the absorption of some essential nutrients and alters the natural bowel flora.

The evidence

The anecdotal evidence suggesting that these drugs can cause candidiasis is overwhelming and there are several references on this subject in medical journals.[4]

Tranquillizers and Irritable Bowel Syndrome/chronic candidiasis
To the writer's knowledge there have been no medical reports of adverse effects on the gastrointestinal system from medium- or long-term use of tranquillizers, but the mass of anecdotal evidence reporting gastrointestinal problems from tranquillizer groups throughout the world cannot be ignored, and no doubt in time there will be scientific research to confirm such findings.

What tranquillizers and sleeping pills do to the gut is unclear but there is no doubt at all that a very high percentage of users develop Irritable Bowel Syndrome and systemic candidiasis, or some manifestation of fungal infections, either during therapy or during withdrawal. The symptoms can persist for many years after complete withdrawal of the drugs. More gastrointestinal problems were reported in people taking lorazepam ('Ativan') than the other drugs in the group such as diazepam ('Valium'). It is known that these drugs block the absorption of zinc so it is possible that they hinder the absorption of other vital nutrients and thus allow the body to become depleted; candida thrives in these circumstances. It could be that the benzodiazepines, in common with the drugs mentioned earlier, raise blood glucose levels thus providing more food for the candida, since many (non-diabetic) users who measured their blood glucose levels found that they were abnormally high after their medication and dropped below normal when the next dose was due. Cemitidine lowers gastric acid secretion and therefore produces an ideal environment for candida growth.

Some tranquillizer users had also been on long-term Cemitidine therapy for symptoms of gastritis caused by withdrawal, but this was only a proportion of those who presented with candidiasis.

Non-drug anti-fungal substances

Garlic – nature's wonder cure

Garlic is an extremely potent fungicide. Its use in the treatment of candida and many other health problems is highly recommended, except of course for people who cannot tolerate it. Its high sulphur content is probably the reason why some people have problems with it. If you know you cannot tolerate anything in the onion family then garlic treatment is probably not for you. If it merely gives you more wind and you don't have other signs of intolerance, such as palpitations, headaches, or muscle pains, just be patient and your digestive system will get used to it.

During the nineteenth century men and women largely turned from the use of natural remedies they had prepared from plants, minerals and animals, to the use of synthetic drugs. Garlic was known by ancient peoples to cure a wide range of ailments: fevers, chest infections, infected wounds, parasitic infection and venomous bites. It was also used for kidney problems and stomach ulcers. The Roman historian Pliny the Elder observed Greek doctors using garlic and recorded:

> It is good for increasing the flow of urine. The best time to eat it is when one is about to drink too much, or when one is drunk. Garlic boiled or roasted is a diuretic, and relaxes the stomach. Garlic causes flatulence, because it stops flatulence.

The last statement may be a reference to what we now know as the homoeopathic principle of like curing like, or it may be that eating foods which cause gas often has the effect of increasing the pressure in the bowel which in effect carries all before it and allows the trapped wind to be expelled.

Modern research confirms that not only did the historical applications of garlic prove correct, but also that it is powerful medicine for much that ails our technologically advanced, polluted, toxic, drug-orientated, twentieth-century world. It has now been found to be antibacterial, anti-fungal, anti-tumour, and to be of great benefit to the circulatory system. It also lowers cholesterol levels. Since it is such a powerful cleanser it detoxifies, eliminating drug residues and environmental pollutants. Chronic cystitis sufferers have found that regular use completely clears their symptoms and obviates the need for antibiotics. Some people find it lifts depression and gives energy. One woman said 'I feel as though I'm on wheels'. This may be because in addition to cleansing the body, it is a useful source of trace minerals such as copper, iron, selenium and zinc.

Garlic is effective in a wide range of bacterial, fungal and parasitic infections. Even the fumes from freshly pressed garlic can kill fungus grown on a Petri dish in the laboratory.

In the gut, unlike antibiotics, it kills off the harmful organisms, protects against the toxins produced, and encourages the growth of helpful organisms. In addition it aids digestion.

Dr Susan Minney writes:

If the active antibacterial compounds within the garlic powder were isolated then, weight for weight, their potency would be very similar to most antibiotics.

Garlic has distinct advantages over antibiotics in that its side effects are very minimal or absent and also that bacteria have not shown any tendency to become resistant to dried garlic.

In summary, the use of dried garlic should be seriously considered in the treatment, or part treatment, of sub-acute, non-life threatening or chronic bacterial infections, e.g. sore throats, bronchitis, cystitis, skin infections, boils, gastroenteritis and diarrhoea. It is probable that the use of garlic in life-threatening, acute bacterial diseases will always be secondary to antibiotics.[5]

Using fresh garlic

This is an inexpensive, safe way to treat candida overgrowth. Its drawbacks are the antisocial effects and for some people the taste. If you (or your family) find these too much to bear you can use one of the deodorized commercial preparations but note that the pills must contain the active ingredient *allicin* to be an effective fungicide.

Most garlic pearles have lost this during manufacture.

Crush one clove (a segment of the bulb) and take immediately either mixed with yoghurt, milk, mashed vegetables or in olive oil poured on salad. Wash down with plenty of water. You may feel a burning sensation or slightly sick for a minute but this soon passes and is replaced by a feeling of warmth and, for some, well-being. Do this three times daily with or after food. The fact that the garlic odour can even be noticed on the skin confirms that, in common with one of the television commercials for a certain lager, it reaches parts many other fungicides cannot reach. Incidentally this makes it a good insect repellent.

Garlic can also be usefully absorbed through the skin; garlic rubbed on a baby's feet can be noticed on its breath. Miners used to put fresh cloves of garlic in their clogs to keep them free from chest infections. For a fascinating history of the use of garlic and how to prepare inhalations, and external remedies see *Garlic – Nature's Original Remedy*, by John Blackwood and Stephen Fulder.

Health-food stores stock garlic products but the quality can be variable. 'Garlicin' from BioCare, a biotechnology company who have an active team in the field of garlic research and the capability to produce a consistently high-quality product, can be ordered by post (see Useful Adresses).

The garlic experience

Here are the stories of two people who ignored the pleas of their families and completely cured their symptoms by using fresh garlic.

Julia

Julia was, in her words, 'in a state'. She had recurrent thrush and cystitis, her face was bloated and covered in blemishes. Every few weeks she developed a cold, mouth ulcers or cold sores on her mouth or inside her nose. Her other problems were weight gain and a persistent rash on her upper arms and chest. She had a history of taking street drugs and abusing alcohol but had been drug-free for two years and only drank at the weekends. Her diet was yeast- and sugar-laden and her only exercise was walking to college some fifteen minutes from her home.

Because she had some answers and a plan of action she felt less depressed and after a week on fresh garlic, a clean diet and taking more exercise she could see physical improvements, and her bladder problems had gone. Three weeks later she was greatly improved; she had lost five pounds in weight, the spots on her face had cleared. The itching and burning in the vulva had gone and the discharge was much less. She had been using a douche of two cloves of crushed garlic to a pint of warm water. Straining the garlic water before use avoided 'bits'. She continued taking garlic with occasional lapses for six weeks and kept to her new eating plan. The rash on her arms and chest improved over the months but did not finally clear until she used 'Canestan' cream. Within three months she felt 'a totally new person'. For Julia it was also an exercise in self-assertion, being able to disregard the complaints of the family. Since she had often been told she 'never finished anything' her self-esteem was boosted by the fact that she had completed her treatment.

Julia's story illustrates how discouraging it is to work hard to be drug-free, and then to be confronted by a new set of problems. There is very little information around on what can happen in the body after withdrawal from street drugs or when some medications are reduced or withdrawn.

John

John had suffered from a bowel infection whilst travelling in India a year earlier. Hospital tests had all been negative. He complained of feeling lethargic, bloated, of loss of appetite and more recently of a rash around his genitals. He was vegetarian and did not like sweet foods so his diet needed little adjusting. He was in the middle of a three-week colon cleanse prescribed by a herbalist. This had given him diarrhoea, but he knew that was all to the good. He took three cloves of raw garlic daily and in addition often had it cooked in his meals. He increased the protein in his diet and took yeast-free nutritional supplements. Within a month he felt stronger and whilst he was still bloated he was not so uncomfortable and his appetite had improved. His energy returned and the fungal rash cleared with sea bathing and sunshine.

John's experience highlights the fact that when you are using garlic, the precise nature of the infection does not really matter because it deals with pathogenic bacteria, fungi or parasites. Whether it was a candida overgrowth due to a stressed immune system or whether it was a parasite he had picked up on his travels, garlic effected his cure.

Caprylic Acid

This fatty acid is a component of certain food fats which men and women have included in their diet for centuries.[6] It works selectively to inhibit the growth of yeasts leaving lactobacillus unharmed. It is found in large quantities in breast milk. Commercial preparations are made from coconut oil and are in most health-food stores. 'Mycropryl' (BioCare) is reliable and is also available in junior strength. It is very effective and side-effects are rare, but it should not be used by persons with gastritis, gastric ulceration or intestinal ulceration. Citricidal (New Nutrition) is an excellent product.

Herbs

One of the newest anti-fungal, antibacterial, antiparasitic substances which also has some anti-viral activity is made from grapefruit seed extract.

Berberine is present in a number of medicinal plants including goldenseal, oregan grape and barberry. These plants have been used in the treatment of diarrhoea in India and in traditional Chinese medicine for three thousand years. Artemisia Annua, another traditional Chinese herb, is used for intestinal parasites. A formula containing all the above substances is marketed under the name 'Eradicin Forte'. 'Tricycline' is a similar product (available from BioCare). These products are very effective and can be used with other products such as caprylic acid or other anti-fungals. They should not be used during pregnancy. This is the only contraindication issued by the manufacturers but it is to be wondered whether the grapefruit seed extract would give rise to symptoms in citrus-intolerant persons. You might need a letter or prescription from your doctor (prescriptions for supplements on the NHS, page 76) before you can order these preparations.

The science of probiotics

This is the use of live bacterial supplements to kill off harmful bacteria in the gut and restore health. The benefits of lactobacillus acidophilus have been known since the beginning of the century and have become a routine part of nutritional and preventative medicine. Nutritionists believe that many degenerative diseases begin with disturbances in the gut bacteria. After cleansing, the colon needs to be recolonized with helpful bacteria. Health-food shops stock bacterial supplements but these cannot always be relied upon to contain live bacteria. It is better to order from a company (BioCare) whose products have this guarantee. If you are milk intolerant you will need to look for a milk-free strain.

Live yoghurt will provide you with some helpful organisms but it is unlikely that this will be enough to recolonize the gut if you have a candida problem.

Homoeopathy and Candida

Elisabeth Edmundson is a trained nurse and midwife and a registered homoeopathic practitioner. She has had an interest in candida problems for many years and uses a combination of homoeopathy, supplements and diet.

Hippocrates stated that he would rather know what sort of person had a disease than what sort of disease a person had. He went on to say:

> A physician who is an honour to his profession is one who has due regard to the seasons of the year and the diseases they produce; to the states of the wind peculiar to each country and the quality of its waters; who looks carefully at the locality of towns and of surrounding country, whether they are low or high, hot or cold, wet or dry; who moreover takes note of the diet and regimen of the inhabitants, and, in a word, of *all* the causes that may produce disorder in the animal economy.

First, it is necessary to discuss the principles of homoeopathy in order to understand how we arrive at the appropriate remedy. It is this remedy which strengthens the fighting ability of the body toward disease, in this case candidiasis.

Conventional medicine treats the symptoms which the person presents. On the other hand, the homoeopath treats the *whole* person. For instance, take an arbitrary figure of five patients with acne. The orthodox practitioner will treat all of them similarly, whereas the homoeopath, because he or she is treating the *person* as opposed to the symptoms, may end up prescribing different remedies for each of them. Although they all have acne, the disease has manifested through different medical backgrounds with varying causes. The homoeopath takes a detailed history, looking at the uniqueness of the individual. The purpose of this close scrutiny is to elicit enough information to paint a picture, thus enabling a remedy selection appropriate to the totality of the person's symptoms. The potency of the remedy is then selected, which ideally matches the dynamic plane of the disease at that time. When the remedy and potency have been chosen, this is called the *similimum*, and when the patient picture matches the remedy picture progress is almost guaranteed.

Principles

- The foundation of homoeopathy is *similia similibus curantur*: 'Like shall be cured by like' or 'That which makes sick shall heal'. Samuel Hahnemann, the founder of homoeopathy, states that the matching remedy for a disease is a substance which in a healthy person produces the same symptoms as displayed in the sick person.

- *The single remedy*. All the symptoms are arranged in order of importance, and the remedy is given. The principle of the single remedy treating the whole person is in sharp contrast to the allopathic system where often multiple drugs are prescribed at one time.

- *The minimum dose*. Very minute doses of the selected remedy are administered. Hahnemann discovered that by reducing dosages unwanted aggravations were reduced and yet the remedies were still effective. He went on to develop a system of diluting remedies to a point where not a single molecule of the original substance is present, only its energy pattern. He called this process of repeated dilution along with succussion or shaking, *potentization*. (In the old days succussion took place on the family Bible, whereas nowadays machines are used.) Apparently it is in the succussion that curative properties are released and believed to work on the deeper subtler spheres of the human being, so the higher the the potency the smaller the amount of the medicinal substance present in solution.

- *Provings*. Substances used are from animal, vegetable and mineral sources. Their potentially healing properties are tested on healthy persons where there is no risk of results being tainted by a disease picture. Hahnemann in fact dosed himself with Peruvian Bark and eventually 'tipped over' into full-blown symptoms of malaria. When he stopped taking the medication he became well again. Today this substance is used homoeo-pathically in the treatment of malaria.

How does it work?

At the centre of homoeopathy is the concept of the Vital Force.

World philosophies recognize this unseen energy – Prana, Ch'i, Bio-energy. When the body manifests symptoms they are seen as the visible expression of the disturbed Vital Force. Orthodox medicine sees symptoms as evidence of a morbid process that must be eradicated or suppressed, and it puts great store by the study of pathological change, chemical disturbances, bacteria and viruses, which leads to treatments directed against them. Homoeopathy, on the other hand, views illness as a dynamic disturbance of the Vital Force and it is *that* which must be restored to full functional harmony.

Symptoms are simply the *result* of a disease and not its cause. In health the Vital Force keeps the 'clocks wound', whereas in sickness the clocks 'wind down' because the immunity is weakened and symptoms develop. When the remedy is given, this stimulates the immune system into action again.

How will this help our patient with candidiasis?

In my experience this problem is best tackled using dietary means, with suitable supplements (recommended is the Cantrol Pack available from Health Plus Ltd – see Useful Addresses) concomitantly with the selected homoeopathic remedy. It is important to stress that although the candidiasis can be fairly easily treated, underlying causes must be addressed: for example, repeated antibiotics for recurring sore throats – homoeopathy will reduce that predisposition.

Case 1: 32-year-old female, L. A.

Complained of:
- halitosis (teeth checked – musty odour);
- bloating and belching after meals;
- prone to sore throats – frequent antibiotics;
- craves sweets and chocolates;
- allergies to lanolin and topical alcohol;
- strong light induces migraine;
- no energy or stamina;
- poor memory;
- muscle weakness;
- poor, unrefreshing sleep.

She had been on the pill for 9 years.

Progress: Marked improvement after one month. Required further treatment for three months. Homoeopathic remedies effectively strengthened her immune system. She married in six months and discontinued the pill. Prolonged exposure to the pill and frequent courses of antibiotics I felt were the culprits.

Case 2: 23-year-old female, J. H.

Complained of:
- Severe depression for 2 years – prescribed antidepressants by psychiatrist;
- feels alone, forsaken, suicidal, weepy, worse in morning;
- 'as if seeing things out of focus';
- 'as if out of touch with reality';
- 'no middle moods';
- 'fears something will happen';
- easily stressed;
- poor sleep;
- recurrent tonsillitis, treated with antibiotics – always 'low' afterwards;
- profound energy lack – wondered if had ME, severe PMT.

Progress: Drugs slowly reduced under supervision. After one month a dramatic improvement mentally. It took nine months for her to be symptom-free, and now this patient is in control of her life.

Homoeopathy is a powerful and necessary facet of candida treatment, because it treats the cause – why the patient becomes susceptible initially.

Elizabeth Edmundson

Essential oils

Before discussing the use of essential oils it must be said that whilst many of them can safely be included in self-help care, they are powerful substances and some are toxic. It is therefore important to follow the instructions of a qualified aromatherapist or use only the oils recommended in aromatherapy books. There are some excellent ones on the market which give clear instructions on choosing and mixing oils for everyday problems such as tension, headaches, indigestion, lethargy, anxiety, depression and so on. They can also be of great value in home beauty treatments. Please note: beauty therapists are only trained to use the oils to promote relaxation and for skin care; they are not trained to use them for specific medicinal effects (aromatherapy).

61

The medicinal value of distilled oil from plants, fruit, wood and resins has been known for thousands of years. During the past thirty years there has been a resurgence of interest in their use and medical research has confirmed that they are not merely pleasant smells which relax or stimulate the body, but that they have great value in alleviating or curing a wide range of physical and emotional conditions. They can be administered through the skin, through inhalation or orally.

When mixed with a base or carrier oil they are absorbed through the fatty tissue of the body during massage. A twenty-minute soak in the bath in warm water with a few drops of oil allows the same penetration. When inhaled from a tissue, in hot water or from an oil burner, the vapours enter a primitive part of the brain called the lymbic system. Tranquillizers also use this part of the brain.

Except where a book clearly states that the oils can be taken orally, for example one drop of peppermint oil in a tumbler of warm water for the relief of wind, they should not be taken internally unless prescribed by a qualified aromatherapist.

Many of the oils have bactericidal and fungicidal properties, but the most important one for candida is tea tree.

Tea tree oil for candida and other problems

For thousands of years the Bundjalung Aborigines of Northern New South Wales have valued the healing properties of the tree *Melaleuca alternifolia*. There are over three hundred varieties of the tea tree but only one produces the medicinal oil. Research shows[7] that pure tea tree oil is an extremely complex substance containing at least forty-eight organic compounds which work together in synergy to produce maximum healing benefit.

The first European to collect samples of the leaves was Joseph Banks in 1770. About the same time Captain Cook's sailors made a 'spicy and refreshing tea' from the leaves to replace the tea they had brought from England – hence the name.

In 1922 an Australian chemist conducted experiments and announced his results to the Royal Society of New South Wales. He discovered the very high antiseptic power of the oil: thirteen times stronger than the carbolic acid which was used at the time (it is now known that it is four times stronger than modern household disinfectants). His findings prompted more research and in

January, 1930, under the heading of 'A New Australian Germicide', the editor of the *Medical Journal of Australia* reported on the use of the oil in general practice.

The results obtained in a variety of conditions when first tried were most encouraging, a striking feature being that it dissolved pus and left the surfaces of infected wounds clean, so that its germicidal action became more effective without any apparent damage to the tissues.

In 1930 the British Medical Journal stated: 'The oil is a powerful disinfectant, but it is non-poisonous and non-irritant, and has been used successfully in a very wide range of septic conditions.'

Although it was found to be effective in so many conditions, including fungal skin problems, demand outstripped production and synthetic germicides were developed. With the advent of 'miracle drugs' (starting with synthetic penicillin) the value of tea tree was overlooked.

In the 1970s there was a renewal of interest in the oil and now over ten tonnes are produced annually in Australia. It is now available in a wide range of products world-wide.

Tea tree oil can effectively treat a great number of ailments, due to its healing and infection fighting properties, including athlete's foot, toenail infection, acne and dermatitis, mouth ulcers and cold sores, and a number of other complaints associated with candida and fungal infections. Its value in treating thrush and cystitis is described on page 16. You will find tea tree oil in most stockists of essential oils. 'Thursday Plantation' (see Useful Addresses) is a reliable brand and they also make a range of skin and hair care products and produce an excellent leaflet detailing the uses of tea tree oil.

Notes

1 W. N. Spellacy, 'A review of carbohydrate metabolism and the oral contraceptives', *American Journal of Obstetric Gynecology*, Vol. 104, 1969, pp. 448–60.
2 *Adverse Drug Reaction Bulletin*, No. 121, December 1986.
3 ibid.
4 'Invasive Candidiasis following Cimetidine Therapy', *American Journal of Gastroenterology*, Vol. 1, 1988, pp. 102–3; 'Candida Peritonitis and Cimetidine', *The Lancet*, 30 September 1978.

5 S. Minney, 'Garlic – The Forgotten Aid to Modern Medicine,' *Biomed Newsletter*, Vol. 1, No. 7, 1990.
6 S. Minney, 'Investigation of Anticandidal Activity of Calcium and Magnesium Caprylate', *Biomed Research*, July 1992.
7 G. Swords and C. L. K. Hunter, 'Composition of Australian Tea Tree Oil (Melaleuca alternifolia)', *Journal of Agricultural Food and Chemistry*, Vol. 26, No. 3, 1978.

7
Diet

It is impossible to set out a candida diet which would suit everyone. There are so many approaches to diets for the control of candidiasis that if you have read a few books on the subject you could end up being totally confused. Some practitioners insist on very strict regimes, others say don't worry too much if you are on anti-candida medication, eat what you like (this would seem to be going too far, progress would be slow). Others say keep to a diet and if you have an odd lapse just take an extra dose of your anti-fungal substance. Before you read on and get discouraged by the idea of a restricted diet there are other ways (see p. 29 on desensitization), although remember you are unlikely to recover from any condition if you abuse your body with junk foods, excessive alcohol and so on.

The right diet for you
Your personal choice will be determined obviously by likes and dislikes, the severity of your symptoms, how desperate you are for them to disappear, food intolerances, and how much stress is involved for you in rigid dieting. This chapter will suggest a strict anti-candida diet and a more relaxed eating plan. You might choose to follow diet one for the first three weeks. Very restricted diets for long periods should be avoided not only because of the danger of your intake being nutritionally narrow but also because eating should be a pleasure and not a continual worry. Remember, stress encourages fungal growth.

Diet as a medicine, not a punishment
If you approach the candida diet not as a life sentence to a strange diet, but as a temporary change to improve your health during which, after the first month, you can have the odd lapse and then as your symptoms disappear, look forward to a normal healthy way of eating. A diet laden with refined sugars and fats is dangerous even for those without candida, so it is envisaged that you will never go back to that; it is unlikely that you would want to after you have experienced the difference in your well-being whilst you have been eating healthily. Be kind to yourself, particularly if you have been eating carbohydrates or drinking excessively for comfort. You

might feel anxiety or grief at having to give up your 'security blanket'. So often the cry is 'but I cannot live without bread' – you can, and you will, if it is necessary and if you really want to get better.

The following are guidelines to starve the candida:

- Absolutely fresh foods.
- No refined carbohydrates.
- Restrict unrefined carbohydrates.
- Aim for a diet as low as possible in yeast.
- Avoid or cut down on foods which contain antibiotics or steroids.

Overripe fruit, limp vegetables and bread that has been around for a few days all harbour mould spores. If possible, shop for smaller quantities from stores which have a rapid turnover of produce. Take extra care over storage of food; wash out the bread bin regularly or store bread in fridge. If you are using only very small quantities, slice a loaf as soon as you buy it and freeze it. You can take your ration out daily. It defrosts quickly or can be toasted from frozen.

Diet one: moderate approach

Avoid or cut down on:

- sugar, white or brown,
- treacle, golden syrup,
- molasses, sucrose, glucose dextrose, marmalade, jam;
- white flour and all products made from white flour: cakes, buns, teacakes, biscuits;
- all processesd grains including some prepared breakfast cereals;
- yeasty foods: hard cheese, blue cheese, marmite/vegemite, brewer's yeast or any supplements containing yeast, vinegar and all fermented products;
- alcohol, fizzy drinks, fruit squashes;
- dried fruit;
- tinned fruit in syrup.

Eat

- whole grains: wholegrain bread, pasta, brown rice, any other unrefined grains;

- puffed wheat, puffed rice, shredded wheat – all sugar-free, also sugar-free muesli or homemade muesli;
- meat, poultry, eggs, dairy produce: milk, cream, butter, cottage cheese, soft cheeses, fromage frais, yoghurt – preferably plain or diet;
- fish – fresh or tinned;
- legumes: lentils, peas, beans, chickpeas;
- nuts and seeds;
- spices;
- fresh or dried herbs;
- large quantities of vegetables raw or cooked;
- useful thickeners for soups and stews: arrowroot; grated potatoes; additive-free vegetable stock: marigold, available from health-food stores;
- fresh fruit;
- olive oil, any other vegetable oil, margarine or butter;
- low-sugar jam;
- diet drinks (in moderation);
- fructose (fruit sugar), honey (in moderation);
- dry white wine or spirit with low-sugar mixer or water (in moderation).

Diet two: strict approach

You could use this for three weeks to get a good start, or before starting anti-fungal drugs/substances. This would minimize the die-off symptoms.

Banned

- sugar, white or brown; treacle, golden syrup, molasses, sucrose, glucose dextrose, any product containing sugar;
- white flour and all products made from white flour: cakes, buns, teacakes, biscuits;
- pasta, white rice;
- all prepared breakfast cereals;
- cured products: bacon, kippers, smoked salmon;
- all fermented products, vinegar, pickles, chutney, sauerkraut, tofu, soy sauce;
- alcohol;
- tea, coffee, cocoa, Ovaltine, Horlicks;
- any malted product;

- all dairy produce: milk, cheese, cottage cheese (possible exception of live plain yoghurt);
- mushrooms, truffles;
- dried fruit;
- fresh fruit for first three weeks;
- spices, dried herbs;
- tinned foods;
- artificial sweeteners, diet drinks;
- nuts;
- citric acid;
- cream of tartar.

Allowed

- restricted whole grains: up to 80 gms per day (one small slice of wholegrain bread = 30 gms);
- brown rice, Ryvita, rye bread, rice cakes, oat cakes, whole oats, millet, buckwheat, barley;
- wholewheat pasta, wholewheat noodles, buckwheat pasta;
- free-range chicken, eggs, turkey, duck, rabbit, lamb, venison, fresh fish, shellfish;
- legumes: peas, beans, lentils, chickpeas, etc.;
- seeds: sunflower, sesame, linseed, pumpkin;
- all vegetables (eat mountains of them) raw or cooked;
- sea vegetables;
- well-washed, peeled fruit.

Why some of these foods are banned

All the foods on the formidable 'banned' list either feed candida, or contain additives which chronic sufferers could have intolerances to. The bloom of fruit is mould, and nuts and spices often harbour mould. Some nutritionists ban artificial sweeteners because some of them are made from sugar (Nutrasweet and saccharin are not) and they believe that their inclusion in the diet perpetuates a craving for sugar.

Note. Some lifelong tea and coffee drinkers can abstain without any problems. Others can have what is known as the 'Caffeine Storm'. This is when all the caffeine in the body is mobilized and before it is eliminated it can cause severe headaches, nausea and aches and pains. A cup of tea or coffee usually eases the symptoms within half an hour. If this happens to you phase tea and coffee out gradually.

Sugar

You do not need sugar for energy. On the contrary, it can drain your energy away. It is not only empty calories, it is the food of choice for the candida and it prevents the absorption of essential minerals and vitamins. It also plays havoc with your blood-sugar levels and disrupts the function of your pancreas causing a multitude of unpleasant symptoms including panic attacks. The importance of keeping blood-sugar levels stable has been fully explained in *Coping Successfully with Panic Attacks* by the same author and publisher.

Sugar in tea or coffee should be stopped immediately. You will get used to it eventually and if it makes you cut down on tea and coffee, so much the better. Try not to turn to regular use of artificial sweeteners; this just prolongs the desire for sweet drinks. Occasional use of sweeteners or a diet soft drink can be regarded as a treat. Withdrawal or sugar craving causes some people to abandon the diet. If you feel in danger of doing this use *very small* amounts of fructose, fruit sugar (this looks like sugar and is available from pharmacies and health-food stores), or honey. These do not disturb the pancreas and are less likely to trigger yeast growth. Look for honey from bees which have not been fed sugar. Organic honey is best but there may be brands which are less expensive.

There are some useful yeast-/sugar-free cookbooks on the market. *The Candida Cookbook* by the same author, published by Thorsons, will be out in 1995.

Refined carbohydrates (sugar and starches)

All refined grains and products made from refined grains encourage yeast growth. They have also lost many essential nutrients in processing. Diets high in refined starches are the main cause of the Toxic Colon Syndrome. The starch combines with mucus in the gut and forms a gluey layer which collects on the bowel wall. The effects of this have been described earlier. There is little argument about the inclusion of refined carbohydrates in the diet; most practitioners recommend their avoidance, except perhaps where someone with a wheat intolerance finds white bread, particularly toasted, less of a problem.

Diet drinks

Some people imagine because they are sugar-free (although check labels because some sweeteners are sugar-based – Nutrasweet is not) that it is fine to drink a large bottle of Diet Coke daily. Since you are trying to clean chemicals and additives from your system this does not seem a good idea. All soft drinks contain citric acid. This encourages yeast growth and can also make cystitis sufferers very uncomfortable. You could make your own soft drinks from freshly squeezed fruit juice and carbonated water.

Dairy products

There is a division of opinion on dairy products. Some practitioners recommend them particularly for underweight people and believe lactic acid to be helpful in candida problems; others discourage their use. Dairy products are mucus-forming and it would be well to avoid them if you have chest or catarrhal problems, if you are intolerant to them or if you are on a colon-cleansing programme. Otherwise go by how you feel if you include them.

Eggs

It is a pity that eggs have had such a bad press lately. Egg yolks are rich in essential nutrients and also help to keep the bowel flora healthy.[1] If you are not in a high-risk heart disease group and if they are taken as part of a healthy diet, their cholesterol content is not a problem. People happily include foods which are much higher in cholesterol and additives, and much lower in nutrients, for example, pasties, sausage rolls and hamburgers. A well-cooked egg is a useful addition to the anti-candida diet. Free-range eggs do not contain antibiotics.

Complex or unrefined carbohydrates

Whole grains and products retain all their nutrients and because their fibre content has not been discarded give the stool bulk and stimulate peristalsis (the contractions and movements in the bowel), thereby keeping it clean. Bacteria acting on the cereal fibre prevent fungal growth. Complex carbohydrates are broken down slowly in the body and release a steady flow of glucose into the blood which prevents the 'kangarooing' of blood glucose levels, with its resultant drop in energy and craving for sugary foods.

There is a division of opinion on whether to restrict complex carbohydrates. Some practitioners say eat as much as you wish of any whole grain you can tolerate. Others restrict them, saying that they still encourage fungal growth even if they are unrefined.

Will changing my diet affect me?

It could, particularly if you have been accustomed to a high refined carbohydrates menu. You might experience withdrawal symptoms, including sugar craving. Change of diet and/or the addition of supplements can also produce lethargy and aches and pains in the first few weeks. Be prepared for this and welcome it: it can be the candida dying off or the effect of other toxins being released from the body.

Diet for an inflamed bowel

This is not strictly an anti-candida measure but can be a help to soothe the digestive tract, clean the colon and give the liver and kidneys a rest before you start anti-candida treatment. It is a diet for people whose digestive symptoms have been fully investigated by their doctor.

Savoury

1   Simmer for an hour and a half a large pan of any fresh vegetables, root and green (even lettuce), except those in the onion family, plus parsley or any fresh herb of your choosing. Add marigold stock powder or vegetable stock cubes.

2   Use this stock (but do not eat the vegetables) to cook white rice. Cook the rice well. If you can bear it, it is better to use plenty of stock, give it a long slow cook and take it as a thick soup. If this does not appeal, you can cook it less and have it as separate fluffy grains. Sprinkle with a little rock salt or marigold powder if it is too bland for your taste.

Sweet

Cook white rice with a little rock salt. Have this hot or cold with plain yoghurt and a little honey or apple juice.

Take

1 teaspoon of slippery elm bark (not slippery elm drink with added milk but the pure bark available in whole-food shops), in water, three times daily.

It is also available in tablet form from health-food stores or from GERARD (see Useful Addresses). Isogel from Boots, an inexpensive, soothing bulking agent will have a similar effect although some people say it gives them wind.

Drink

Water (bottled if possible), herb teas or, if you get a headache, one or two cups of weak tea or coffee per day, maximum.

Don't wait for meal times

Eat either the savoury or sweet rice whenever you feel like it all during the day. Do not allow yourself to get hungry. If you are underweight don't continue for any more than two days unless you are managing to eat good quantities. If you are overweight you could continue for seven days – the bathroom scales will please you! You might find it boring but nothing is more boring than the nagging soreness of an inflamed digestive tract.

The value of fresh raw vegetables and fruit

This cannot be overemphasized, not only from a nutritional point of view but also as an aid to digestion, to cleanse your system and for enzyme production. Since these are complex carbohydrates you can eat them freely. Many people who have problems with cooked vegetables can eat them raw without producing symptoms. If you prefer them cooked, eat a small salad before your meal or nibble some vegetables as you prepare them. Remember the keyword is *fresh*; there is a great deal of difference between the juice from a fresh orange and a glass of orange juice from a carton.

An exciting book on the energizing effects of raw foods, sprouting seeds and how to cleanse with vegetable and fruit juices is *Raw Energy* by Leslie and Susannah Kenton (see Further Reading).

Nutritional supplements

Many people have commented that they are bewildered by rows of supplements in health food stores. The following information is a guide to help you choose ones which help to build the immune system. If the choice and dosage differs from those suggested by your doctor or nutritionist be guided by them because they will have more knowledge about your individual needs. If you find you cannot take supplements at the suggested dosages build up to the full dosage slowly or take them two or three times a week if that is all you can manage. Remember that supplements should be regarded as a medicine to correct deficiencies and as such should be taken as a course and not indefinitely unless this has been advised by your doctor or nutritionist. Follow the instructions on the bottle carefully and keep them out of the reach of children.

Penny Davenport, a member of the Register of Nutritional Therapists, has worked as a nutritional adviser for more than ten years, for nine years with a large supplement company and for two years independently. She gives personal and telephone consultations specializing in candida and detoxification problems.

The supplement list recommended to combat candida seems endless, so I have singled out those below which I feel are the most important.

Vitamins

Vitamin A
As beta carotene, 25,00 iu's or 15mg in good quality supplements – this is the same amount.

B complex
Single B vitamins should always be taken with the complex to ensure balance.

Vitamin B 5–500mg
Important for combating stress.

Biotin 800mcg
Prevents the yeast from becoming invasive, often comes with folic acid.

Vitamin C 3–5grams
As a sustained release formula, or in small divided doses, anti-viral and immune boosting.

Minerals

Zinc 15–50 mg
Elemental form, the dose on the label is often higher so check, for immune function.

Selenium 200 mcg

Inhibits free radical damage.

Kelp 2-6 daily

All essential trace minerals, excellent for balancing the thyroid gland, which often contributes to a low immune system.

Magnesium 200mg

Taken in the morning, helps muscle ache and fatigue.

Probiotics

As well as Bifido bacteria and acidophilus, Lactobacillus Salivarius, is newly available, it digests protein molecules that have not been completely digested, a common cause of autotoxicity.

Digesive Enzymes

1-2 with each meal, or as needed. Incompletely digested food causes many problems, there are now a variety of vegetarian formulations, these are often preferred to the animal type, some are in vegetable gelatin.

Anti-parasite

Grapefruit seed concentrated extract. Many candida sufferers are found to have parasites.

Herbs

Garlic

Highly anti-fungal and promotes the growth of probiotic organisms.

Echinacea

Stimulates production of white blood cells.

Combinations

Artemesia, Barberry, Pulsatilla and Zingiber with grapefruit extract, are antibiotic, anti-fungal and anti-parasite.
Chinese herbs like shizandra, acanthopanax and astragalus boost immunity.

Pau d'Arco tea

Boosts the immune system, and strongly anti-fungal.

Essential Fatty Acids

Gamma Linoleic Acid and Evening Primrose Oil 1–4 gms daily, essential to produce balanced hormones, prostaglandins; one function is to keep yeast cells at bay, and to stimulate the immunity gland, the thymus, to produce T Cells.

If you are on a limited income, you must stick to the diet first. It is not expensive – think what you would save on your normal shopping bill: no bread, biscuits, cakes, tea, coffee, sweet drinks, no dairy products, not to mention sweets and chocolate, all of which leaves a lot of room for a variety of vegetables. Never go hungry, eat small meals regularly, and drinking water is important.

As supplements are expensive it is important to know which ones to choose and ways of being economical. Vitamin C is essential, the powder is the cheapest, and plain ascorbic acid is under £10 for 200 to 250 grams. Buffered with minerals, it costs a little extra. Herbs are always economical and making a tisane is simple. Capsules and tablets cost more, but generally less than £10 for a three to four weeks' supply. As they boost the immune system and are anti-fungal, and in some cases anti-parasitic as well, the new combinations can be useful. With probiotics try the cheaper ones first to see if they work for you, but sometimes it makes more sense to take less of a quality concentrated form, but find the one that works for you. Garlic is important, eat as much as you can, but if this is socially impossible there are odourless varieties, but as they are highly concentrated they are more costly. A good all-round food concentrate that gives a wide range of essential nutrients is a fresh water algae called Chlorella, and a month's supply should be less than £10. Many sympathetic practitioners dispense supplies in weekly packs, so it is always worth asking. If you cannot find one or your local health shop does not stock the items you want, there are excellent mail order companies who also specialize in giving advice. For details of these and the suppliers of the other nutritional supplements mentioned here, see Useful Addresses.

Penny Davenport

Nutritional supplements on the NHS

Can my doctor prescribe nutritional supplements?

The answer is yes. The procedure is explained in full in an excellent leaflet 'NHS prescribing of nutritional supplements' produced by the Nutrition Associates.

Nutrition Associates emphasize that any preparation can be prescribed by a GP as long as it is not on the 'blacklist' and in the case of actual and potential vitamin deficiency, vitamins are regarded as drugs for prescribing purposes.

Many doctors believe supplements cannot be supplied on prescription, but the chairman of the regulating body has said there should be: 'no problem about prescribing vitamins for proven deficiencies on a normal prescription form. It is a medical decision based on proven fact, and no-one would argue with any such prescription.'

Nutritional supplements can therefore be prescribed when there are proven nutritional deficiencies or good clinical evidence of such deficiencies. Unfortunately, many of the vitamin and mineral preparations prescribed by GPs are of a formula or a dosage level that makes them unsuitable for nutritional therapy. Vitamins tend to be of too low, and minerals far too high a dose level. Moreover, few of them take account of the need to give a broad range of nutrients to avoid causing secondary deficiencies.

Multiple deficiencies

As it is well established that single vitamin deficiencies seldom exist in isolation, where one or more have been proven others are likely to exist.

Since vitamins usually have to be taken in combination to achieve their desired and optimal effects, well-formulated, good-quality multinutrient preparations are usually needed to back up specific supplements of vitamins being used to treat proven nutritional deficiencies.

Unfortunately, many of the best vitamin and mineral preparations are produced or supplied by companies other than those with which chemists are used to dealing. The preparations need to be hypo-allergenic, as many preparations contain hidden ingredients (such as flavourings, colourings, preservatives, fillers and excipients), synthetic or natural, to which many people can be allergic. In order to ensure the right quantity and quality of nutritional preparations, it is often necessary for the GP to write the firm's name on the prescription. Nature's Best, Lamberts, and Quest (now Phoenix), are all recommended, as are Throne, Klaire and Cardiovascular Research products, for example, (although these last three would have to be supplied to the chemist in the UK by Nutrition Associates, who are the sole agents for these products made by American firms).

As many patients are hard put to afford the extra expense of buying preparations themselves, it is preferable that whenever possible GPs will co-operate by prescribing them. If you, or your GP, need further advice you can contact Nutrition Associates (see Useful Addresses for details).

Diet neurosis

Practitioners helping people with candida and allergy problems have increasingly become aware of what I have called 'candida/allergy diet neurosis'. Some people (even those under medical supervision) become so obsessed by what they can't eat that the diet becomes very narrow. They become malnourished and this affects the immune and nervous systems, with the result that there have been hospital admissions for nervous breakdowns and anorexia.

Relax, be balanced, have the odd treat, rotate your foods, watch your weight and above all understand that dietary adjustments are a temporary medicine to clean the digestive tract and help your immune system. What is the point of ending up with a pristine digestive tract if you have endangered your health in other ways?

Notes

1 Carl C. Pfeiffer, *Mental and Elemental Nutrients* (Keats Publishing Inc., Connecticut, 1975), p. 264.

8
Looking After Yourself

Taking care of your general health is a vital part of the anti-candida programme. Stimulating the circulation and lymphatic system by exercise and getting plenty of fresh air and daylight should be taken very seriously. Early nights are also essential.

Exercise

Exercise is an important part of recovery from most conditions and it is often hard to convince people of this. They seem to think because they feel low they should be as inactive as possible. If you do not have a fever, inflamed muscles, or any condition likely to be adversely affected by exercise, such as ME (check with your doctor if you are unsure), then *move*; you will delay your recovery if you don't.

It would be unwise to start vigorous activities if you have been sitting around for months. Build up the amount of exercise slowly. You will see below why it is so important.

Inactivity affects the circulation and consequently organic function, for example, the digestion, becomes sluggish; this causes constipation. Muscles are also affected, not only by lack of nourishment, but also by a build-up of crystals which are formed from the waste products of digestion. This can cause generalized aches and pains and local tender spots. If you don't move, the crystals cannot be dispersed. Tension also locks these crystals into the muscles; a build-up in the shoulder area can be very painful and, in turn, cause you to move less.

If you do not move the muscles of the neck and shoulders, you restrict the blood supply to the head and give yourself endless problems. You need to ask yourself how much you are holding yourself back by sitting long hours in a car, at a desk or even watching television without moving. The brain can become sluggish, too, and when full circulation is restored symptoms of anxiety and depression can be dramatically relieved. Building simple stretching exercises into your daily life or a brisk walk in your lunchtime break take little time and can be a start, but you have to make more time for exercise if you really want to feel the benefits.

78

The lymphatic system

This is part of the body's defence against disease. A body fluid called lymph, which relies on muscle contraction for its circulation, is carried through a complex network of small vessels which carry cellular refuse on the way. It is then passed into the bloodstream where it is processed. The lymphatic system does not have a pump (unlike the blood circulation which has the heart) and if you don't move then the lymph slows down. The result can be fluid retention and cells which rely on lymph for their nourishment becoming malnourished. Even if you have to stay in bed for some reason you can still help to circulate the lymph by gently squeezing each group of muscles in turn, and rotating the ankles and wrists. Massage can also be very helpful.

Aerobic exercise

Aerobic exercise is, by definition, exercise which utilizes the long, smooth muscles of the upper legs and arms. This muscle pumps blood (and lymphatic fluid) to the heart and liver, and to the lungs for cleansing and oxygenating, thereby boosting the immune system by encouraging regeneration and white blood cell replacement. Aerobic exercise also stimulates the production of serotonin, a sleep precursor, and endorphins, which are pleasure giving and pain relieving. It promotes sleep because muscle growth and cell replacement is a result of exercise, but can only take place during sleep. It strengthens the muscles of the heart and increases the capacity of the lungs.

For aerobic exercise to be effective, it needs to be done for 20 minutes, 3 times a week, at a pace that makes you breathe deeply and hard, but not out of breath. A target heart-rate range must be sustained for 20 minutes. It should be an effort, but not exhausting. Swimming, walking, gentle jogging, running, cycling, step and aerobic classes are all examples of aerobic exercise.

Water therapies

Caution: Consult your doctor before using water treatments if you have heart trouble, raised blood pressure, diabetes, epilepsy or have any condition which might be aggravated by extremes of temperature. If you are on medication, particularly tranquillizers, it is also advisable to check with your doctor.

Sea bathing

The tonic effect of sea bathing is well known but perhaps it is less well known that even walking ankle deep in the sea boosts circulation and can be very soothing for the nervous system. Tension can be discharged through the soles of the feet as they are massaged by the sand – rather like the effect of reflexology.

Hydrotherapy

Hydrotherapy has been used in spas for thousands of years. Treatments include immersing parts of the body in different temperatures as in a Sitzbath – sitting in hot water with the feet in cold for three minutes then reversing for one minute and repeating this procedure several times. The result is quite dramatic: a glowing feeling the whole length of the spine. It also boosts the immune system and circulation in the abdominal organs. It is not easy to do without special plumbing but it can be done at home with a bath, two buckets and a baby bath. It can also be done with two baby baths.

1   Sit in bath of hot water with feet in bucket of cold water. The hot water around the bucket will raise the temperature so keep the water cold with an ice pack or a plastic bottle (about mineral water size) two-thirds full of water which has been frozen. After three minutes get out, lift out cold bucket and change.
2   Sit in baby bath of cold water and put feet in bucket of hot water. After one minute change again.
3   Sit in the hot for another three minutes. Make sure water in bath is still hot. You will not get the same effect with tepid water.
4   Change from sitting in hot to cold at least three times.

This might seem like a lot of effort but the effect is worth it. Alternate hot and brief cold showers are also invigorating but do not give such a dramatic lift.

Mineral baths

Seaweed, mud, herb and essential oil baths all have detoxifying and healing properties and can promote relaxation.

During the past hundred years the popularity of hydrotherapy has waned and people turned away from natural healing methods toward drugs, sometimes with disastrous results. Those who have sought water treatments have often been regarded as cranks. The

80

climate of public opinion could change now owing to the work of Professor Vijay Kakkar, of the Thrombosis Research Institute in London. Even before *The European* (29th April to 2nd May, 1993) had gone to press, news of his findings had flashed around the world and calls from Australia, Canada and Russia for more information jammed the switchboard.

Cold baths (TRHT)

Professor Kakkar's research has shown that thermo-regulatory hydro-therapy strengthens the immune system, boosts testosterone in men, and oestrogen in women (this could help menopausal symptoms), increases the circulation, helps asthma and could prevent thrombosis. A research programme was carried out at the Institute on 5,000 volunteers. In the article, Dr Anne Macintyre, author of *ME: Post-viral Fatigue Syndrome and How to Live with it,* said 'It all makes good sense.' A reduction of the natural killer white blood cells makes it difficult for the immune system to fight infection. 'Cold water would stimulate circulation and the lymph glands, so I can see the logic of what is being put forward.' Professor Kakkar stated 'We are putting a scientific sense into something that is widely practised. This is for the benefit of the people. That is why I wanted to publish it now,' he said. 'But I would strongly urge those interested in this to adhere to the programme and follow the health warnings.'

Note: Since this study finished, information packs are no longer available. You could, however, write to *The European* (Useful Addresses) for a copy of the article (date above) or look it up in your local library.

If cold water is not for you

The skin, in effect, is the largest organ in the body. Whilst the digestive tract and the kidneys are the main organs of excretion the skin also has a very important part to play; it is a great deal more useful than just a waterproof covering which stops us falling apart. If it is kept healthy it can be a wonderful waste-disposal system. It covers such a large area it is worth getting it to work for you.

A fever is Nature's way of helping us to lose toxins through the skin. You can stimulate sweating with some water therapies. Steam baths, saunas and jacuzzis encourage detoxification. Exercises in water or swimming also stimulate the lymphatic system and rid the body of toxins.

Salt baths encourage detoxification and greatly help muscle and joint pains. Add 2 lbs of salt or three cups' full of Epsom salts to a comfortably hot bath and lie in it for twenty minutes; add hot water as it cools. If you drink a pint of hot water with the juice of half a lemon and a teaspoonful of honey, or peppermint tea, whilst you soak it will further encourage sweating. An ice-pack or cold flannel on the forehead might make you feel more comfortable.

If you wrap up in warm towels or a cotton sheet and get into a warm bed you should perspire freely and sleep well. If you have to bathe during the day finish with a cold shower and rest for half an hour. You could do this three times weekly.

You could have a foot bath whilst reading or watching the television. It helps to stimulate the circulation and ease aching feet. Use bowls of hot and cold water alternately, staying two minutes in each; carry on for about twenty minutes. If you wish you could add one cup of salt or half a cup of Epsom salts to the hot water and an ice pack to the cold. When you have finished, wrap the feet in a towel and rest.

Skin brushing

For people who hate exercise, this is a good way to stimulate the lymphatic system. It involves brushing all over with a natural bristle brush for about ten minutes before your shower or bath. Start with the soles of the feet and work on all areas except broken skin, the face, neck and breasts. It can be boring but the results are worth it. In addition to eliminating toxins, because circulation is increased, it will also improve the texture of your skin. Boots, Green Farm and the Body Shop have skin brushes, or you might have an old hairbrush that would do the job; wash it carefully.

Swimming

Swimming stimulates the immune system and has been shown to elevate mood. Allergy sufferers may be affected by chlorinated water.

Light, sun, air

Daylight is necessary for normal brain functioning (see 'Seasonal Affective Disorder', *Coping with Anxiety and Depression*, by the same author and *Daylight Robbery* by Damien Downing – details of both in Further Reading), and for the regulation of the sleep–wake cycle; staying indoors when you are depressed or ill can only compound your problems. Even if you are severely agoraphobic you could sit at an open window without your glasses; do this for a minimum of twenty minutes daily in the brightest part of the day.

Sunlight kills bacteria and fungus on the skin. Short exposure to ultraviolet light, either from the sun or a sunbed can be of great benefit to fungal skin infections. Baking in the sun for hours or overdoing sunbed treatments ages the skin and can lead to skin cancer. Frequent exposure for short periods has other beneficial effects, including the production of Vitamin D. We also look healthier after a little sun and this increases feelings of well-being.

Exposure to fresh air also kills fungus. Unless they actually have chest problems, it is often difficult to convince people of the benefits of good breathing habits, and even harder to impress upon them the dangers of continually filling the lungs with stale air. Candida sufferers should avoid being in dank, mouldy places such as cellars and damp rooms and going out when the weather is warm and moist. At such times the air is laden with fungal spores. They should, as has been said in the allergy section, avoid paint fumes, being near photocopiers and other chemical pollutants.

Electrical pollution

The immune system can be affected by working environments contaminated by low-level radiation from electrical equipment and from an overload of positive ions. If ventilation is poor and we walk on synthetic carpets, wear synthetic clothes and are surrounded by plastic furniture, we are unlikely to feel good at the end of the day. In cities, stale air can be trapped between tall buildings. Electrically polluted air can be the cause not only of respiratory problems but also of headaches, irritability, digestive problems and depression.

Particles in the air around us, ions, are electrically charged, positive and negative. There should be a balance between the two. We breathe in these particles and absorb them through the skin. If the air is overloaded with positively charged particles it can have a powerful effect on the nervous system. The brain overproduces a chemical called *serotonin* and this can produce nasal congestion, lethargy, feeling sticky (not the same feeling as being too hot) and swollen. The oppressive feeling before an electrical storm best describes this, a restless feeling, being 'under the weather'.

Negative ions have a tonic effect on the nervous system and

reduce histamine levels in the blood. As any allergy sufferer knows, histamine is strongly associated with unpleasant feelings. The benefits of negative ionization are becoming widely known not only for cleaning the air, killing bacteria and viruses, but also as a treatment for asthma, bronchitis, migraine, burns, scalds and wounds. Candida sufferers, particularly if they have allergies, would do well to buy an ionizer to use in the bedroom. They are also available for use in a car and can be found in most department stores. After a thunderstorm the air is negatively charged; it smells fresh and we experience 'the calm after the storm', our energy returns and our mood improves. The air by the sea, waterfalls and flowing water, even by the shower, is also negatively charged and can produce a feeling of well-being. Some people are more affected by this than others, in the same way that some people are irritable and restless when the moon is full and others do not notice it. At full moon, the positively charged layer of the ionosphere, air and particles which absorb harmful radiation from the sun, is pushed nearer the earth, thus increasing the number of positive ions in the air we breathe.

You cannot overdo negative ions; there is no maximum dosage; you can breathe in as many as you like. Some people have ionizers in every room. If you have one in your sitting-room don't forget to put it by your bed at night where it will help you to have a restful night.

The state of the electromagnetic field

We are electrical beings: our hearts, brains, muscles and nerves all produce a subtle form of electricity and this discharges around our bodies and forms an electromagnetic field. All living things are surrounded by this field, and in the 1930s a Russian called Kirlian developed a form of photography which clearly showed this field.

The influence on the whole being – body, mind and soul – of the electromagnetic field (also known as an 'aura') is dismissed by many scientists and considered merely to be mystical nonsense. This is unfortunate since some scientists believe that disease manifests in the electromagnetic field *before* physical symptoms appear. This can be demonstrated by Kirlian photography.

One of the first people to study what he called the L-fields or the fields of life and how they affect health, was Harold Saxon Burr, of Yale University Medical School. Dr Robert O. Becker, author of

The Body Electric, a leading modern researcher on electromagnetic pollution, believes that human-made electromagnetic fields from power lines and electrical appliances can cause depression, a depressed immune system and other health problems. Working on the electromagnetic field could be the medicine of the future, the prevention and treatment of illness through balancing areas of low energy. This knowledge is not new, and similarities can be found in ancient forms of healing. Because of the work of American nurse Dolores Kreiger, a technique which clears and energizes the electro-magnetic field is taught in some nursing schools; it is known as therapeutic touch. She describes this in her book *Therapeutic Touch: How To Use Your Hands to Help or Heal,* published by Prentice-Hall, New Jersey. Janet Macrae, one of Dolores Kreiger's students, has written a simple book which anyone could use, called *Therapeutic Touch: A Practical Guide,* published by Knopf. My only reservation about this book is: do not worry if you do not feel the different qualities of the energies she describes when you are working either on yourself or other people: what you feel is what *you* feel; don't try to fit that into the experience of someone else. Your hands are unique. Both of these books can be ordered from good bookstores.

Can I feel my own electrical field?

Only 1 per cent of people can't – try it. You might have to try on a few occasions before you can be sure, but the more you practise, the more sensitive your hands will become. There are several ways to build up the energy in your hands before you use them. Here is a simple one I saw in a Julie Soskin workshop. Breathe in slowly and visualize yourself being filled with Universal Energy, Prana, Ch'i or whatever you wish to call it.

Increasing the energy between your hands

1 Hold your arms out in front of you, raising one about a foot above the other.
2 Clench and release the fists rapidly for about fifteen seconds.
3 Lower the raised hand and raise the other; repeat the fist clenching and releasing.
4 Keeping the arms out in front; repeat 2 and 3.
5 Relax the shoulders; point the fingers upwards as if you were going to clap. Make a 'concertina' movement with the hands in and out, just a few inches but do not bring the palms into contact.

You will feel a resistance or a feeling of pressure, heat or tingling between your hands. Some people say they feel as if there is foam rubber between their palms, others describe feelings of tingling, throbbing or pulling.

Using your hands to clear the electromagnetic field

Now that your hands are energized you can use them to clear positive ions from your immediate environment, relieve headaches and nasal congestion, increase relaxation, and ease discomfort in muscles and joints.

1 Rub your feet and massage under the arch for about a minute. If your feet are very tense take a little longer over it, then place them flat on the floor if sitting.
2 Sit relaxed or lie on the floor or bed; slow down your breathing.
3 Close your eyes and imagine yourself totally well and peaceful. If you cannot get this image, give yourself the command, 'I am totally well and peaceful', and imagine a pure white light is entering your head, filling your body and coming out from your fingers and palms. Reach up beyond your head and stroke about three to four inches above your body just as though you were touching it; down over your face, neck, chest and abdomen, and then sweep the hands to either side of the body. This is important because you need to take the congestion clear of your body. You will feel prickling or heat in your hands as you pick up congestion. You can just flick this off as though you are shaking water from your hands.
4 Continue stroking for about ten minutes or until your arms feel tired.
5 Now, still imagining you are filled with white light and seeing it coming from your hands, hold them over your abdomen and imagine your digestive tract and all your internal organs becoming healthy and vitalized.

Increasing energy in selected areas

In this part of the exercise you are sending energy to an area of discomfort, perhaps an aching knee or bloated abdomen. You may feel heat or cold and possibly rumblings in your gut. Don't be surprised if it makes loud noises. This is just a sign that you are relaxing. As you practise this you will get a feeling of being 'finished'. That is the only way to describe the sensation of an area having taken enough energy. You might also have noticed your nose feeling less congested or your sinuses making popping noises when you were working around your head. You can transfer energy in the same way to any aching muscles or joints that you can reach. Clearing congestion from the field also helps to cool a fever, ease itching and reduce swelling.

Many people get very enthusiastic about therapeutic touch and are keen to use it to help others. This is certainly to be encouraged but not before you are well and have learned more about it. There are people who teach this technique, which is sometimes called 'auric massage'.

The inner child, the spirit

This might appear to be a strange conclusion to a book on a parasitic yeast, but since I believe that total health is dependent on the harmony of body, mind and spirit, I felt the need to include, with humility, the little I have learned in my own emotional and spiritual struggle.

Parasitic emotions

Negative feelings about ourselves, lack of self-worth, lack of self-love, anger, failure to see our place in the world, and fears, particularly the fear of the death of our physical bodies, can continually eat away at our life force, preventing us living in the here and now, and disrupting our lives as much as yeast overgrowths in the gut, or any other physical problem.

Where do these feelings come from and why do we hang onto them? They come from our life experience (beginning prenatally), and we are often reluctant to give them up because in order to do this they have to be confronted. Most of us shy away from this out of fear, or we lack the insight to see that these suppressed emotions are causing us any problems. We use tension, hyperventilation (over-breathing), physical illness, addictions to alcohol, drugs, sleep, power, work, TV, sport, gambling, searching for relationships, money, even compulsive talking and use of the telephone – any number of mechanisms – to contain the fear and emptiness of the inner child, thus building up the wall of neurosis (see my book, *Coping with Anxiety and Depression*). 'Neurosis' should not be used as a put-down word to describe what we consider odd behaviour in someone else; it simply means a reaction to trapped pain, an inner child, and consequently a soul, or whatever you will call your higher self, longing to be acknowledged, loved and brought together to make a whole person, a person who is centred, peaceful with themselves, their Creator, and the world about them. A helpful book on connecting with your inner child is *Healing Your Aloneness* by Erika J. Chopich and Margaret Paul.

How can I love myself?

First, wake up, be open to the possibility that you are not meeting your needs – you are crying inside – and find a counsellor, psychotherapist or even a friend to support you whilst you explore this; realize that self-love takes a great deal of practice and be aware that it is very different from narcissism and selfishness. M. Scott Peck in his book *The Road Less Travelled* covers this subject with wisdom and love.

Questions to ask yourself

- Am I crying inside?
- Am I lonely, even in company?
- Am I using mechanisms like hyperventilation and addiction to alcohol?
- Am I judgemental?
- Do I continually criticize the behaviour of others?
- Do I blame others, my life circumstances, the world, for my feelings?
- Am I always looking for a tomorrow that never comes?
- Do I continually look to others for approval?
- Have I taken on board the negative feelings people from my past and present – mother/father/siblings/teachers/employers/ partners – have about me?
- Do I feel their feelings about me to be unjust and untrue and yet reinforce their accusations by refusing to give them up?
- Am I afraid?
- Am I too afraid of fear itself to face why I am afraid?
- Am I afraid to express anger?
- Does my anger come out in inappropriate places – on the people I know will take my anger and still love me, or on strangers where I do not risk losing love?
- Am I afraid to love – even myself?

- Am I puzzled by my behaviour towards others; is it how I really want to behave?
- Do I feel totally unlovable?

Integrating the inner child, the adult, the Spirit

Even if we are born into loving, secure backgrounds it is very unlikely that our needs will be correctly interpreted and met, and after all it is rather unreasonable of us to expect that this should be so. I believe that we ask for our life experience, as harsh and bewildering as it might be, in order for our souls to progress. I do not believe that suffering is redemptive: my understanding is that God, full of unconditional love, is ever with us on our chosen path, suffers when we suffer, and is joyful when we find peace and fulfilment. What is more I believe we are here to love and to learn; that is what we take with us into the next world, and if we can be happy whilst we journey this is just how it was intended. What loving father would want it any other way? Although *I* consider myself a Christian, many people would disagree, since I believe that it is impossible to evolve spiritually in one lifetime and that we are reincarnated many times in order to do this. I believe that the Scriptures, whilst full of truth and beauty, have been 'cut and pasted' by human beings, particularly by the Church, in an attempt to become more powerful, so that some essential truths have been lost.

Religiosity against spirituality

Exchange unprofitable religious speculations for actual God-contact. Clear your mind of dogmatic theological debris.

Lahiri Mahasaya (1828–95)

If you are happy into your chosen religion and feel at peace with yourself, with God, and with your fellow human beings, then you will not need these pages. If on the other hand you feel empty, longing for spiritual peace, and confused, then look beyond your own religious backyard and be open to good in all religions and philosophies; when you are ready your teacher will appear, books you need will 'drop into your lap', you will hear wisdom and find unconditional Love in unlikely places; furthermore you will know these truths and you will recognize that Love.

Further Reading

Chapter 2

Maggie Tisserand, *Aromatherapy for Women,* Thorsons 1985.

Chapter 3

Dr Jonathan Brostoff and Linda Gamlin, *Food Allergy and Intolerance,* Bloomsbury 1989.

Harvey and Marilyn Diamond, *Fit For Life,* Bantam 1987.

M. Katahan, *The Food Rotation Diet,* Bantam 1986.

Amy Magrath, *One Man's Poison – The 'Glucose' Factor* (£6.60 incl. p&p, available from Cirrus Associates – see Useful Addresses). A unique story: one mother's struggle to identify the Glucose factor in carbohydrate which turned her children from unhealthy 'devils' into healthy 'angels'.

Dr Keith Mumby, *The Food Allergy Plan,* Unwin 1985.

Barbara Paterson, *The Allergy Connection,* Thorsons 1985.

Ellen Rothera, *Perhaps It's An Allergy,* Food and Chemical Allergy Association 1988.

Shirley Trickett, *Irritable Bowel Syndrome and Diverticulosis,* new edition, Thorsons 1999.

Celia Wright, *The Wright Diet,* Grafton 1986.

Chapter 4

Cystitis

Angela Kilmartin, *Understanding Cystitis: The Complete Self Help Guide,* Arrow 1989; *Cystitis,* Thorsons 1994; *Sexual Cystitis,* Arrow 1988. Video: *Overcoming Cystitis* (£10.99 incl. p&p from Kilmartin Video Ltd., PO Box 217, Walton-on-Thames, Surrey KT12 3YF.)

ME

Dr Belinda Dawes and Dr Damien Downing, *Why ME?,* Grafton 1989.

Dr B. Dawes, *ME Formula,* a supplement programme available from Lamberts Healthcare Limited, 1 Lamberts Road, Tunbridge Wells TN2 3EQ (01892 513 116/01892 534 574).

FURTHER READING

Dr Ann MacIntire, *ME Post Viral Fatigue Syndrome and How to Live With It,* Thorsons (second edition), 1992.

Mike Franklin and Jane Sullivan, *ME: What is it? How to Get Better,* Random Century, 1989.

Chapter 6

John Blackwood and Stephen Fulder, *Garlic – Nature's Original Remedy,* Javelin 1986.

Chapter 7

Leslie and Susanna Kenton, *Raw Energy,* Arrow 1984.

Shirley Trickett, *The Candida Cookbook,* Thorsons 1995.

Chapter 8

Ericka J. Chopich and Margaret Paul, *Healing Your Aloneness: Finding Love and Wholeness Through Your Inner-Child,* Harper and Row 1990.

Damien Downing, *Daylight Robbery: The Importance of Sunlight to Health,* Arrow 1988.

Shirley Trickett, *Coping with Anxiety and Depression,* Sheldon 1989.

Useful Addresses

Abbey Brook Cactus Nursery
Dept. CP., Baicowell Road, Matlock, Derbyshire DE4 2QJ
Suppliers of *cactus peruvianus,* which is used to absorb low-level radiation.

Action Against Allergy (AAA)
43 The Downs, London SW20
AAA provides an information service on all aspects of allergy and allergy-related illness, which is free to everyone. Supporting members get a Newsletter three times a year and a postal lending library. AAA can supply GPs with the names and addresses of specialist allergy doctors. It also runs a talk-line network which puts sufferers in touch with others through the NHS and itself initiates and supports research. Please enclose s.a.e. (9" x 6") for further information.

Allergy Testing (North-East Area)
Hazel White-Cooper, Homoeopathic Practitioner, 18 Wilmington Close, Tudor Grange, Kenton Bank Foot, Newcastle-upon-Tyne NE3 2SF
Please send SAE for details.

Auric Healthcheck, Healing Crystals
Keith Thompson, 10 Olive Street, Sunderland, Tyne & Wear
Tel. 0191 510 1322

BioCare Ltd
54 Northfield Road, Norton, Birmingham B30 1JH
Tel. 0121 433 3727
Wide range of nutritional supplements for candida control and allergies, including Probiotics, GLA, Mycopryl, and children's formula.

British Holistic Medical Association
179 Gloucester Place, London NW1 6DX

British Society for Nutritional Medicine
Stone House, 9 Weymouth Street, London W1N 3FF
Tel. 0171 436 8532

Cirrus Associates
Food and Environmental Consultancy
Peter G. Cambell B.Sc. Cert Ed FIFST
Little Hintock, Magna, Gillingham, Dorset SP8 5EW
Tel. 01747 838165

Colonic International Association
26 Sea Road, Boscombe, Bournemouth, Dorset BH5 1DF

The Complete Hormone Clinic
Dr Andrew Wright, 57 Chorley New Road, Bolton, Lancs BL1 4QR
Tel. 01204 366101
Dr Wright is trained in orthodox and alternative medicine, and
has a great interest in chronic fatigue, allergies and candida.

Liz Edmundson
Candida Treatment and Homoeopathy
18 Wilmington Close, Tudor Grange, Kenton Bank Foot,
Newcastle-upon-Tyne NE3 2SF
Please send SAE for details.

The European
Orbit House, 5 New Fetter Lane, London EC4A 1AP

Family Health and Nutrition
PO Box 38, Crowborough, Sussex TW6 2YP

Federation of Aromatherapists
46 Dalkeith Road, London SE21

Michael Franklin
1 Squitchey Lane, Apartment 4, Oxford OX2 7LB
Tel. 01865 511357
Trained nutritionist with a special interest in chronic fatigue syndrome, candida and allergies.

G&G Food Supplies
175 London Road, East Grinstead, West Sussex
Tel. 01342 3230 16
Suppliers of Probiotics and Sublinguals.

GERARD
Gerard House Ltd, Wickham Road, Bournemouth, Dorset

Jackie Habgood
Swindon candida, allergy and ME group
40 Priors Hill, Wroughton, Swindon SN4 0RW
Tel. 01793 813 493

Jo Hampton
45 Wainfleet Road, Skegness PE25 3QT
Tel. 01754 768 336
Suppliers of Earthdust candida formula.

Health Plus Ltd
PO Box 86, Seaford, East Sussex BN25 4ZW
Tel. 01323 492 096
Suppliers of the Cantrol Pack of supplements.

Higher Nature
Burwash Common, East Sussex TN19 7LX
Tel. 01435 883964 (team of qualified nutritionists able to give advice); 01435 882880 (mail order). Fax 01435 883720
Dedicated to providing a comprehensive nutritional service. The quality of supplements is excellent, and their 'Nutrition and Beyond' offprints are well worth the 30p price. Higher Nature offer a reliable service for candida/allergy testing, and also have an outstanding range of skin care products (Annemarie Borlind). They make regular contributions of supplements and money to refugees and those in nutritional need.

Hyperactive Children's Support Group
59 Meadowside, Angmering, W. Sussex BN16 4BW

IBS Network
c/o Centre for Human Nutrition, Northern General Hospital, Sheffield S5 7AU
Run by IBS (Irritable Bowel Syndrome) sufferers for IBS sufferers. It offers a quarterly newsletter, *Gut Reaction*, self-help groups, and a 'Can't wait' card. Membership costs £3-£6 p.a. depending on income. For further information send s.a.e.

Institute of Allergy Therapists
Donald M. Harrison, Ffynnonwen, Llangwyrfon, Aberystwyth,
Dyfed SY23 4EY
The Institute maintains a register of practitioners and provides a
referral service for the general public.

Labscan
Biomedical Screening Service
Silver Birches, Private Road, Rodborough Common, Stroud,
Gloucs GL5 5BY
Tel. 01435 873446/873668   Fax. 01435 878588
Labscan is an independent laboratory established to provide a
non-invasive, simple to use, comprehensive diagnostic service for
nutritionists and other practitioners who wish to determine the
ecological status of their patient's intestinal tract.

Larkhall Green Farm
Putney Bridge Road, London SW15
Tel. 0181 874 1130
Supplies Pau d' Arco tea, Caprylic acid.

Life Tool Holdings Ltd (Relaxation aids)
Meridian House, Roe Street, Congleton, Cheshire CW12 1PG
Tel. 01260 282000.   Fax 01260 282001
This firm has two new electronic medical machines. They work
with two ear clips at the press of a button. One reduces anxiety,
improves concentration, lifts depression and aids sleep (Alpha-Stim
SCS) and the other does the same and also treats pain via probes
(Alpha-Stim 100). For £4.95 you can try the Alpha-Stim SCS for a
month without obligation to buy. It is a safe and effective treatment.

ME Action Campaign
PO Box 1126, London W3 0RY

ME Association
PO Box 8, Stanford Le Hope, Essex SS17 8EX
Enclose s.a.e. for information about ME.

National Institute of Medical Herbalists
PO Box 3, Winchester, Hants SO22 6RB

National Society for Research into Allergy
PO Box 45, Hinckley, Leicestershire LE10 1JY
Information on allergy and details of support groups and contacts.

New Nutrition (Penny Davenport)
Woodlands, London Road, Battle, East Sussex TN33 0LP
Tel. 01424 774103
Many people are now seeking natural ways to cleanse the
digestive system from the effects of drugs and careless eating
habits and also to build up the nervous and immune systems
with vitamins and minerals. It is essential to have expert advice
on this. New Nutrition is staffed by experienced nutritionists.
Advice is available via a natural health hotline, a health letter
service, a computer-assisted CARE programme and personal
consultants. They offer seminars on nutrition, special diets,
natural health and skin care. Membership costs £5 per year and
includes telephone advice on supplements and a magazine
three times a year. They charge £3 if you write for advice on
health problems.

Nutrition Associates
Caltres House, Lysander Close, Clifton Moorgate, York YO3 0XB
Medical practice: candida/allergy testing, nutritional profiles.

Nutriscene
28 The Precinct, Rainham, Kent
Tel. 01634 362 267
Supplies herbal combinations, including those to curb candida,
detoxify mercury from fillings and combat geopathic stress.

The Radionics Association
Goose Green, Deddington, Nr Banbury OX15 0SZ
I can personally recommend (as can many of my clients and readers) radionics, a little known alternative approach. It is useful in
a wide variety of conditions. For a practitioner in your area contact the above address.

The Sanford Clinic
15 Lake Road North, Roath Park, Cardiff CF2 5QA
Tel. 01222 747507

Society for Environmental Therapy
3 Atherton Street, Ipswich, Suffolk IP4 2LD

Thursday Plantation
Illingworths, York House, York Street, Bradford BD8 0HR
Tel. 01274 488 511

Wholefood, Organically Grown Produce
24 Paddington Street, London W1DM 4DR

Note for readers in the United States

The nutritional suppliers mentioned in this list are willing to mail their products to the US. The same or similar products can be obtained from American Interplexus Inc., 6620 So 192nd Place, J-105 Kent, WA98032, USA.

Index

INDEX

herbs 57, 74–5, 75
homoeopathy 27, 53, 58–61
hormones 10, 13, 14–15, 32, 43
hygiene 16–17, 20, 33–4

illness 1
immune system 5, 8, 10: food
    intolerance and 28
insomnia 6
ionization 83–4

laxatives 52
lifestyle 3
lymphatic system 79

ME (Myalgic Encephalomyelitis) 41–2,
    49, 81
medical history 11
men 20–2
menopause 14–15
minerals 73–4, 75, 76–7
mood swings 6
moulds 66, 68
mouth 5, 23
'Mycropryl' 57

National Health Service: nutritional
    supplements from 76–7
'Nystatin' 13, 14

Pau d'Arco 47, 49
penises 21, 45–6
pill (contraceptive) 10, 14, 51
pityriasis rosacea 46–8
PMT 17
pollution 1, 34, 83–4
pregnancy 10
probiotics 57–8, 74, 75
psoriasis 44

psychological symptoms 6, 12, 17; case
    histories of 60–1; food intolerance
    and 24

Reiter's syndrome 21
religion 89

sex 11
skin 42–4, 46–8; brushing 82; contact
    dermatitis 21; rashes 5, 21; soreness
    and itching of 48–9; *see also* acne
soy products 25–7
spirit; inner child 3, 89; negative
    emotions and 87–9; religion and 89
steroids 1, 10, 51
stress 1, 10
sugar 32, 69; *see also* diet
sunlight 82–3

tea tree oil 16, 17, 33, 43, 62–3
thrush 15–16; in babies 18; in men 21
Trichomonas vaginalis 15
'Tricycline' 57

urethritis 21
urinary tract 10, 21, 24; cystitis and
    39–41

vaginitis 15
vitamins 37, 73, 75, 76–7; cystitis and
    39; sun and 83

water therapies 15, 79–82
weight control 32–3
women 14–20; cystitis and 40

yeast 8, 49
yoghurt 16, 57–8

zinc 43, 44